D0569874

STRETCHING
FOR ATHLETICS

Pat Croce, LPT, ATC

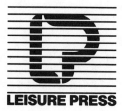

LEISURE PRESS

NEW YORK

A publication of Leisure Press
597 Fifth Ave., New York, New York 10017
Copyright © 1984 by Pasquale Croce, Jr.
All rights reserved. Printed in the U.S.A.

ISBN 88011-119-4
Library of Congress No. 83-80859
First Edition: First Printing 1981
Second Edition: First Printing 1983

Cover Design: Tanya Edgar
Cover and Text Photos: Peter Zinner
Book Design and Production: H&C Custom Publishing Co., Inc.,
Emeryville, California

Charts on pp. 120-123 reprinted by permission from
Dorland's Illustrated Medical Dictionary, 26th edition,
Philadelphia, W.B. Saunders Co., 1981.

I wish to acknowledge with thanks the following for their assist-ance in the preparation of this book: Jim Brennan *and my wife,* Diane, *who posed for demonstration pictures;* Tone Up, Inc. *for the use of their facility; and* Janice Reeder *for her energetic help in writing, editing, and typing the finished product.*

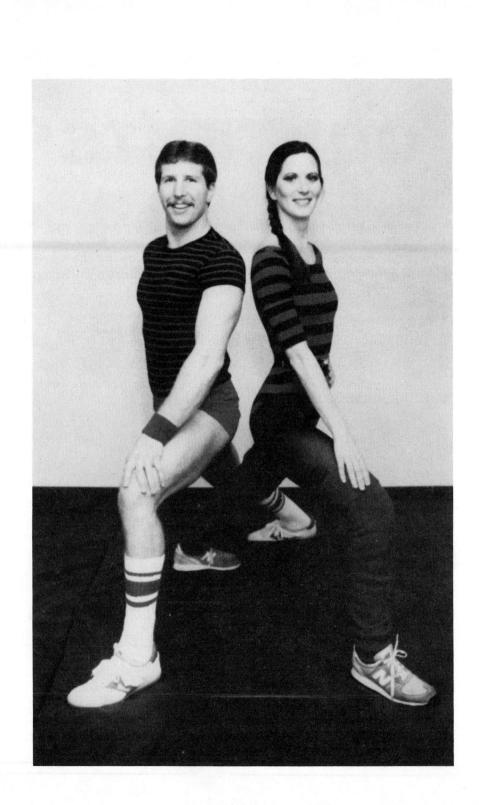

CONTENTS

Introduction

I'm an athlete. I run, I strength train, I play racquetball, and I hold a black belt in karate.

I also stretch every day.

As an athlete, I see the value of stretching in my ability to resist injury. As a physical therapist and athletic trainer, I see the need for stretching in athletes who are hurt because they're out of shape.

Athletes out of shape? It occurs all too often in both amateur and professional competition. Athletes may demand more of their bodies, but like most people they've somehow forgotten the instinct to stretch. And an instinct it is, one just as natural as breathing.

Animals stretch without thinking. So do babies, who stretch as they wake, even before they open their eyes. With no conscious understanding as to why they stretch, they stretch, nevertheless.

As we mature, stretching becomes more a conscious choice than an instinct. And consciously, many of us choose not to stretch. It may be healthy, it may exercise our muscles, it may prevent painful injuries. But as is so aptly expressed in the Life Cereal commercials, we tend to avoid what is good for us. Somehow, we grow up with the conclusion that if something is healthy, it must be unpleasant.

Well, athlete, it's time to wise up. Stretching not only is good for you, it also feels good. Stretching isn't difficult, it's easy. It isn't time consuming, it takes just a few minutes a day. Stretching is affordable, no fancy equipment is required. Stretching can be performed anywhere, at any time.

Best of all, stretching is a wonderful alternative to being sidelined with an injury. If you're serious about sports, your winning efforts must begin well before competition. Your greatest challenge is not the athletes you face but the body you live in every day. Be that body's teammate, not its opponent. Feed it well, provide it with sleep, and regularly stretch the muscles and other connecting tissues it uses to follow you through every waking and resting moment of your life.

If you consciously choose to stop breathing or eating, you know what the results are going to be. Your body can't exist without the nutrients it derives from oxygen and food. To prevent the predictable, you breathe and eat. Unstretched muscles also react in a predictable fashion. They lose the ability to absorb the oxygen and nutrients they require to function. Slowly, they atrophy. Then muscle fibers die. When you need them to compete, the muscles aren't there; or else they're so shriveled that your efforts end in injury.

"Ignorance is bliss," or so goes the saying. For an infant, ignorance results in instinctive stretching. But for you as an athlete, ignorance only leads to sore muscles, repeated attempts at rehabilitation, and the nagging doubt as to whether sports are worth the pain.

Long ago, I learned that the stretching instinct I lost could be replaced with a conscious knowledge of the value and need for stretching.

Stretching For Athletes will provide you that knowledge. Read each chapter carefully, follow the instructions, and perform the exercises properly. Then consciously choose to stretch everyday. And be an athlete to the best of your ability.

Pat Croce, LPT, ATC

1

Stretching's 5 W's

Stretching is so basic that it takes just one letter of the alphabet to describe all its properties.

Why Stretch?

Stretching is good for you; and when you stretch properly, it feels great, too. Your muscles are designed to be long, flexible and lean. In that condition they allow you the range of motion needed for easy, pain-free movement. When you're under stress, your muscles involuntarily contract, creating additional tension. More than any medication, stretching is an excellent tension remedy. It's also cheaper. Stretching relaxes your muscles, and the contractions disappear. As your muscles relax, so do you. Although your source of stress may still exist, a good stretch can help you withstand the tension.

Who Should Stretch?

Someone is spreading a rumor that stretching is only for athletes. Don't believe it. Athletes demand more from their muscles and thus are more likely to be injured. However, everyone, athlete or not, needs to stretch. Muscles are necessary for more than just athletics. You need them for sitting, you need them for shopping, you even use them as you sleep.

Don't make the mistake of listening to rumors. Respond to reality. Stretch.

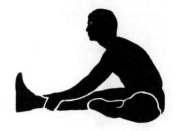

Where Should You Stretch?

Stretching isn't limited by location. You can stretch anywhere. Stretch at home, stretch at work, stretch in stores. It doesn't have to be obvious. You can stretch any muscle group without causing a single raised eyebrow.   Better yet, if you're out in public, attract a little attention. Your own sense of good health might give others the message that stretching is good for them, too.

When Should You Stretch

Athletes must stretch before and after every workout. But *daily* stretching is fundamental to anyone's interest in a well-toned body. As you read *Stretching For Athletics*, the exercises you find will provide the foundation for your own great daily stretch.

Beyond your everyday stretching, however, stretches can be performed at any opportune moment. Stretch when you awake and before you go to sleep. Stretch when you're stiff, stretch if you're tense. Do you like t.v.? Stretch while you're watching it. If you're a reader, try stretching more than your eyes.

With Whom Should I Stretch?

Stretching your muscles won't tone up someone else's body, but peer pressure and group support can mean the difference between neglecting your stretching and sticking to it. Stretching is primarily a singular activity. But if stretching by yourself is boring, for your body's sake, stretch with someone else.

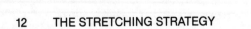

2

The Stretching Strategy

Every successful athlete knows the key to victory is a winning game plan.

Stretching is no different. It, too, demands a basic strategy that can mean the difference between health or harm.

Strategies may differ from sport to sport, but a stretching strategy is the same for everyone. It's simple, it's easy to follow, it makes sense. Best of all, it prevents the kind of injuries that all too often shorten a talented athlete's career.

Here's the strategy.

Stretch daily.

Take your time. Stretch slowly.

Repeat each exercise before moving on to the next one.

Easy does it. Relax as you stretch.

Try not to bounce.

Concentrate on smooth, regular breathing.

Hold each position for 10-20 seconds.

Stretch daily.

When it comes to stretching muscles, gravity is stiff competition. What you work to make flexible, gravity works to contract. If you fail to stretch daily, gravity wins. Long, lean muscles become short, squat, and prone to injury.

Don't be a loser. Stretch every day!

Take your time. Stretch slowly.

Don't underestimate the strength of your muscles. Make a fist. Feel the strength? Flex your bicep. Feel the strength? Contracted muscles are like brick walls — strong, rigid, unyielding. But muscles must also be flexible; or else, like a wall, they will break when enough force is applied against them.

In your body, that force is generated whenever you stretch too quickly. As you stretch, the momentum of your action helps carry muscles to their full range of motion. Slow, controlled momentum increases flexibility without diminishing muscle strength. Sharp, uncontrolled momentum can jerk your muscles beyond their capacity. Yanked by such force, they weaken and break — just like a wall.

To prevent injury, stretch slowly. Control your movements, don't let them control you.

Repeat each exercise before moving on to the next stretch.

When you first perform a stretching exercise, it's a little like sticking your toes in the water. Uncertain of the temperature, you're cautious at first. So you test the water. The first time you stretch, you cautiously test your capability to perform the exercise without stress or pain. Once aware of your limitations, you comfortably can repeat the exercise. This time, however, you stretch a little bit further, thereby increasing your flexiblility.

Easy does it. Relax as you stretch.

When you're tense, your muscles are tense. And tight muscles are difficult to stretch. Relaxed muscles, on the other hand, more easily extend to their full range of motion. So before you stretch, relax.

Try not to bounce.

Bouncing has a similar effect on your muscles as does stretching too quickly. The uncontrolled momentum pulls muscles sharply, forcing them to strain beyond their stretching capacity. Whenever you bounce, you risk the chance of microtears in your muscle fibers. Such an injury can cause so much pain that you'll avoid exercising for several days. Once you return to stretching, your muscles will have lost some of their flexibility. Inflexible muscles are injury-prone, and continued bouncing will only aggravate the situation.

Concentrate on smooth, regular breathing.

Easy breathing is relaxed breathing. When you're relaxed, so are your muscles. And as I've said, relaxed muscles are more flexible. Many athletes make the mistake of holding their breaths while they're holding a stretch. If you hold your breath, you deprive your muscles of the oxygen they need to function. Anoxic (without oxygen) muscles quickly react by developing sharp, painful contractions known as cramps.

To avoid cramps, breathe. To avoid tension, breathe smoothly and regularly.

Hold each position for 10-20 seconds.

Stretching is an education for your muscles. As you stretch, they're learning new extensions of their range of motion capabilities. Within each muscle fiber is a structure called a spindle. Like a spindle on a spinning wheel, your spindles hold your muscle fibers in the position in which you stretch them. Since the purpose of stretching is to extend your range of motion, you must allow your muscles the chance to "learn" the new extension and then to maintain that position on their spindles.

Learning takes time, so give your muscles 10-20 seconds to reeducate themselves.

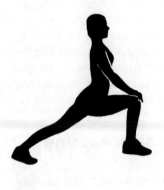

3

The Fundamental Stretch

To reword an old cliche, "A stretch a day keeps the injuries away." Trite? Maybe. True? Yes. Daily stretching is as important to good health as balanced meals and the right amount of sleep.

When you eat or sleep improperly, your body suffers. Lack of stretching creates equally poor results. Every day that you neglect to stretch, your muscles atrophy. Long, lean tissues become short, squat, and inflexible. When you need them to work, your muscles strain; then they tear.

The best prevention for such injuries is a series of eleven exercises called the Fundamental Stretch. Performed daily, they serve as the basis for good muscle health. And, as workers of every major muscle group, they're the primary reason why athletes committed to stretching are injured less often and heal more quickly.

Like other exercises, each Fundamental Stretch exercise must be performed properly in order to be effective. Poor stretching is just as bad as no stretching at all. Follow the directions carefully. The exercises should be undertaken in sequence and each held for 20 seconds. Do each exercise twice before progressing to the next one.

The entire series requires just ten minutes a day.

If you participate in specific sports, you may wish on those days to perform other stretches *in addition to* the Fundamental Stretch. But even when you're inactive athletically, don't neglect the Fundamental Stretch. It's a solid foundation for a flexible body; so start building.

CANNONBALL (Low Back, Neck Extensors)

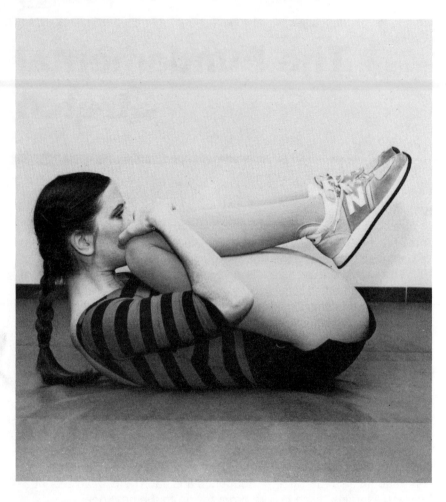

Lie flat on your back. Bend your knees, and place your feet flat on the floor. Grab your knees with your hands, and slowly pull your knees to your chest. At the same time, curl your head to your knees.

SPREAD EAGLE (Groin)

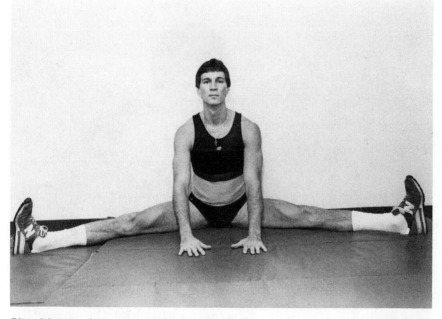

Sit with your legs spread wide. Slowly lean forward, keeping your legs straight.

FIGURE FOUR (Hamstrings)

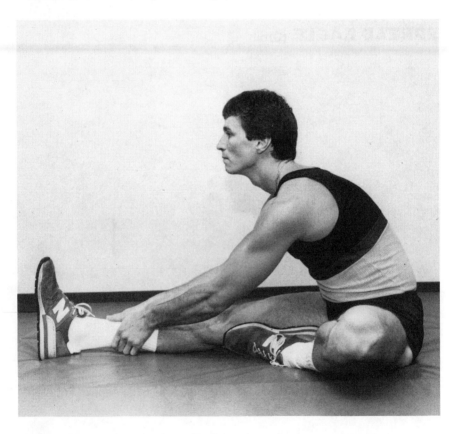

Sit with your right leg straight. Bend your left leg so that your left foot slightly touches the inside of the right thigh. Slowly bend forward at the hips, and try to touch your chin to your right foot. Then reverse leg positions, and repeat the stretch.

PRETZEL (Trunk Rotators, Neck Rotators)

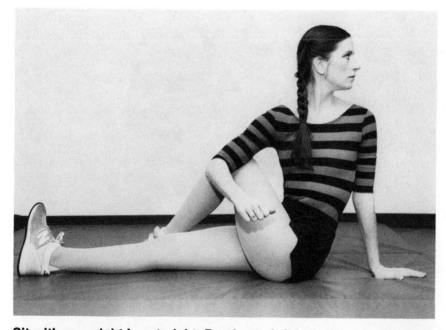

Sit with your right leg straight. Bend your left leg over your right leg, and rest your left foot flat on the floor on the outside of your right knee. Touch your right elbow to the outside of your left knee. Place your left hand on the floor behind you. Then slowly look over your left shoulder, and rotate your trunk to the left. At the same time, apply counter-pressure with your right elbow against your left knee. Reverse leg positions, and stretch to the other side.

ALTAR BOY (Quadriceps, Shins)

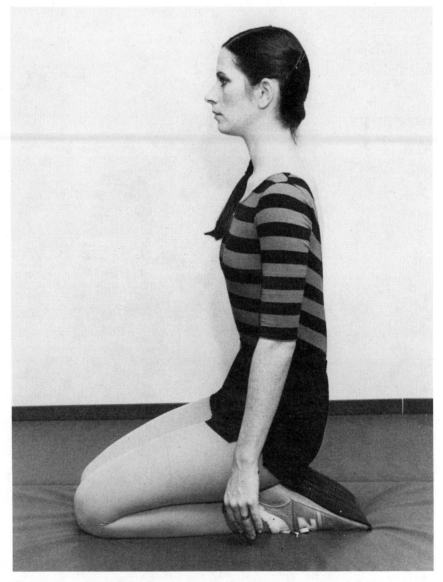

Kneel with the tops of your feet flat on the floor. Slowly sit back on your heels.
*Note: If you have knee problems, don't bend your knees into this position.

FENCER (Hip Flexor)

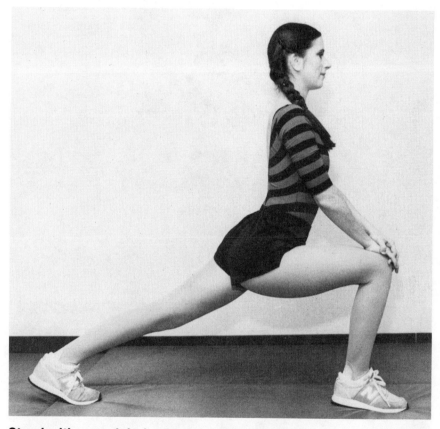

Stand with your right leg bent far enough forward so that your right knee is directly over your right ankle. Straighten your left leg, and raise it on the ball of your left foot. Slowly lower your hips, keeping your back straight. Reverse leg positions, and stretch the other leg.

LEANING TOWER A (Calves)

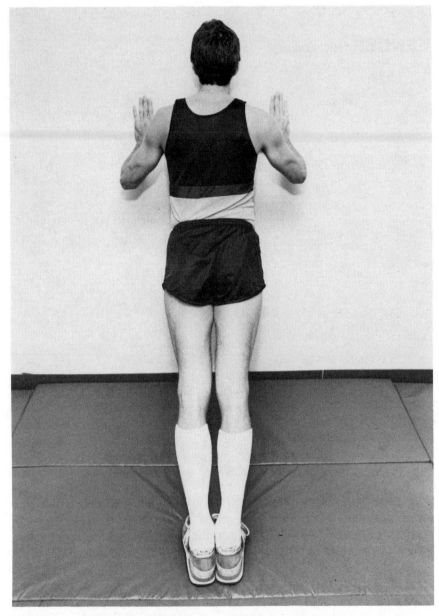

a) Stand facing a wall. Straighten your legs, and place your heels flat on the floor. Using your arms for support, slowly lean forward at the hips.

LEANING TOWER B (Calves)

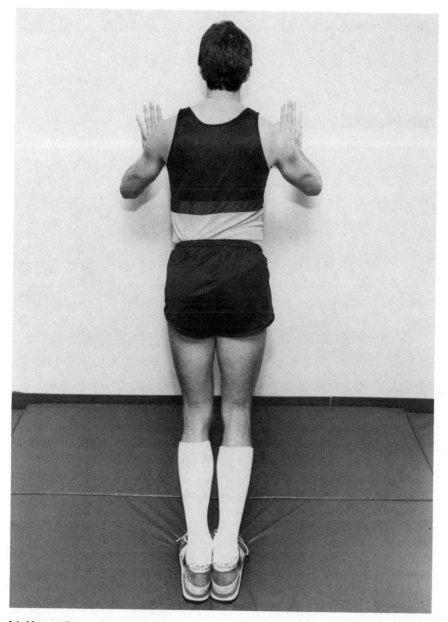

b) Keep the same position as in a. But instead of your hips, slowly bend forward at the knees. Be sure to keep your heels flat on the floor.

AIRPLANE (Chest)

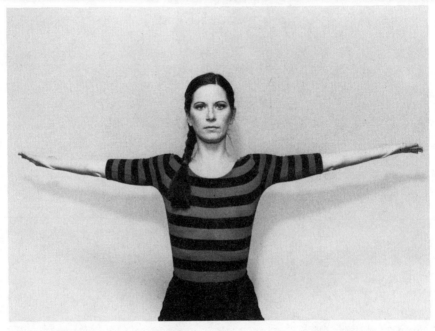

Stand with your arms straight out and at shoulder height. Turn your palms up, and slowly pull your arms back.

PILLAR (Biceps, Latissimus, Wrist Flexors)

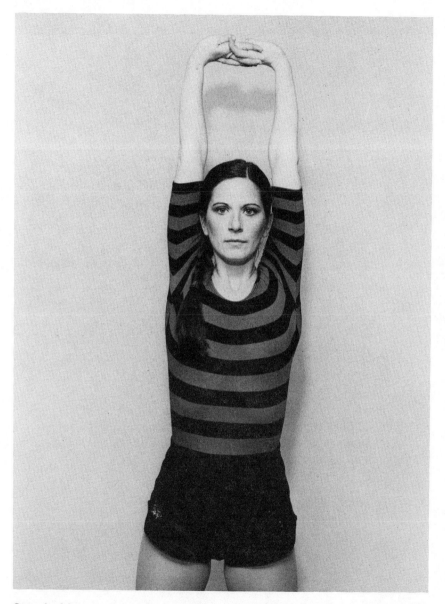

Stand with your arms above your head and with your fingers interlaced.
Straighten your arms, then turn your palms forward and up. Slowly pull
your arms back.

CHICKEN WING (Triceps)

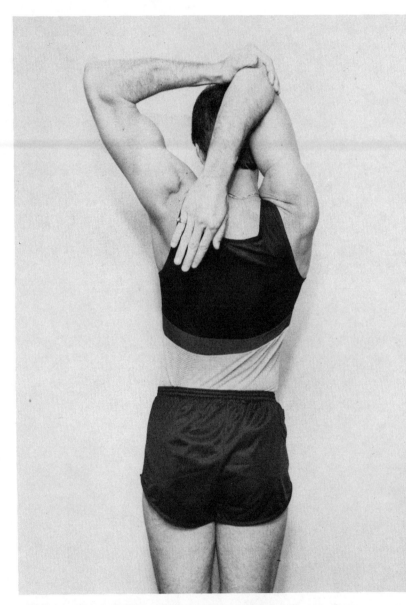

Stand with your right arm bent behind your head. Grasp your right elbow with your left hand, and slowly pull the elbow away from your head. Reverse arm positions, and stretch your other arm.

TEACUP (Rib Cage, Neck Flexors)

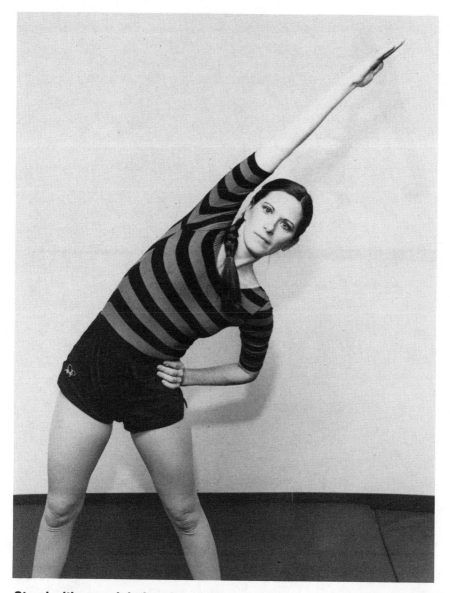

Stand with your right hand straight above your head and with your left hand resting on your left hip. Slowly bend to your left, and pull your right arm over your head. Reverse arm positions, and stretch to the other side.

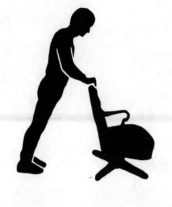

4

Specific Sport Stretches

In any sport, the muscles most likely to be injured are those most often used. If soccer is your game, your legs are at greatest risk. Your arms get a workout if you swim or play golf.

Hard working muscles need extra power and strength to do the job and remain injury free. That power and strength comes from stretching. So on the days you participate in a specific sport, pay special attention to the muscles on which you're making the biggest demands. Remember, neglected muscles tend to get injured. Stretching is the best prevention.

"More stretching?" you ask. You bet. Although the Fundamental Stretch satisfies general flexibility needs, specific sport stretches supply the necessary supplements for times when you're athletically most active. Don't skip the Fundamental Stretch, however. Just add the six stretches listed for the sport you play in Tables 4-1 to 4-16. If your sport isn't listed, choose the exercises listed in a sport that work the same muscles as your sport.

You'll notice that some of the specific sport stretches are part of the Fundamental Stretch. That repetition is what your muscles need to carry them through the demands you place on them. Don't skip a stretch because you've performed it already. What helps your muscles is worth repeating.

Each of the six specific sport stretches should be held for ten seconds. Do each exercise twice before moving on to the next stretch. For ease of motion, perform them in the order they appear.

The entire group will take two minutes.

For the best results, stretch for two minutes as a warm-up prior to athletics and for two minutes as a cool-down after you've finished playing. Warming up heats your muscles, which—like taffy—are stiff when cold and flexible when heated. As a cool-down, stretching readjusts your muscle temperature to its pre-exercise state. Cool-down stretching also rids your body of lactic acid, an exercise by-product that causes cramping and soreness.

Between the Fundamental Stretch and the specific sport stretches, you'll devote only 14 minutes on active days to muscle health. The best athletes think of those 14 minutes as an investment, not a sacrifice. Once you see the results in yourself, you'll understand their point of view.

EXERCISE \ SPORT	Baseball/Softball	Basketball	Bicycling	Dance	Football	Golf	Jogging	Karate	Racquetball/Squash	Skiing	Soccer	Swimming/Rowing	Tennis	Volleyball	Wrestling
Fundamental Stretches	•	•	•	•	•	•	•	•	•	•	•	•	•	•	•
Windshield Wipers	•											•			
Twine	•											•			
Fencer	•	•	•		•	•	•	•		•				•	
Leaning Tower	•	•	•				•		•	•	•		•	•	
Figure Four	•	•	•	•	•		•	•	•	•	•		•	•	
Pretzel	•			•	•	•		•		•					•
Cannonball		•	•	•	•	•	•			•	•				•
Spread Eagle		•	•	•			•	•	•	•			•	•	•
Altar Boy			•	•		•	•			•	•	•			
Pillar		•		•	•			•				•	•	•	•
Airplane				•				•				•	•		•
Teacup					•										•
Criss Cross					•										
Can Opener							•								
Chicken Wing									•				•	•	
Leaning Chair		•												•	

Table 4-1. Listing of recommended specific sport stretches.

BASEBALL/SOFTBALL

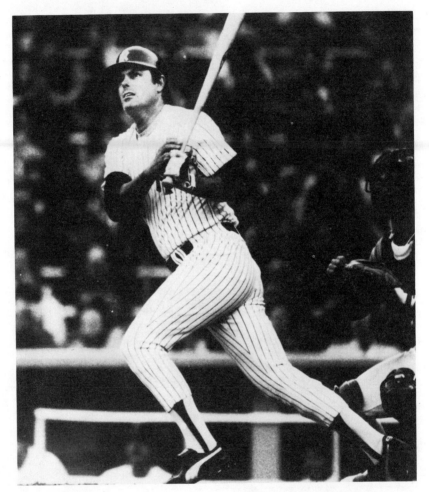

Exercises	Muscle/Area Stretched
1. Windshield Wipers	Neck Rotators
2. Twine	Shoulder Rotators
3. Fencer	Hip Flexors
4. Leaning Tower	Calves
5. Figure Four	Hamstrings
6. Pretzel	Trunk Rotators, Neck Rotators

TABLE 4-2. Specific stretches for baseball and softball.

BASKETBALL

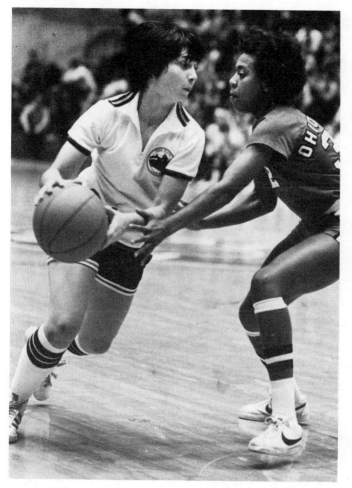

Exercise	Muscle/Area Stretched
1. Leaning Chair	Wrist Flexors
2. Figure Four	Hamstrings
3. Spread Eagle	Groin
4. Fencer	Hip Flexors
5. Pillar	Biceps, Latissimus, Wrist Flexors
6. Leaning Tower	Calves

TABLE 4-3. Specific stretches for basketball.

BICYCLING

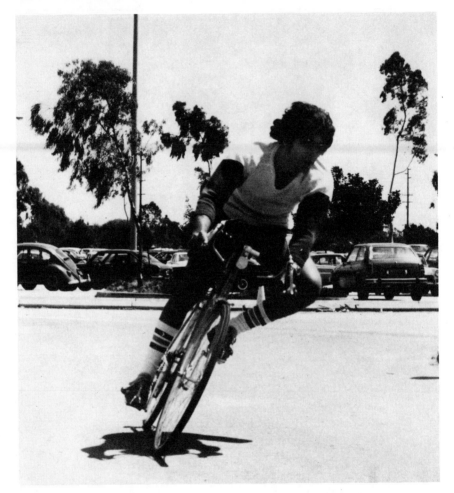

Exercises	Muscle/Area Stretched
1. Cannonball	Low Back, Neck Extensors
2. Spread Eagle	Groin
3. Figure Four	Hamstrings
4. Altar Boy	Quadriceps, Shins
5. Fencer	Hip Flexors
6. Leaning Tower	Calves

TABLE 4-4. Specific stretches for bicycling.

DANCE

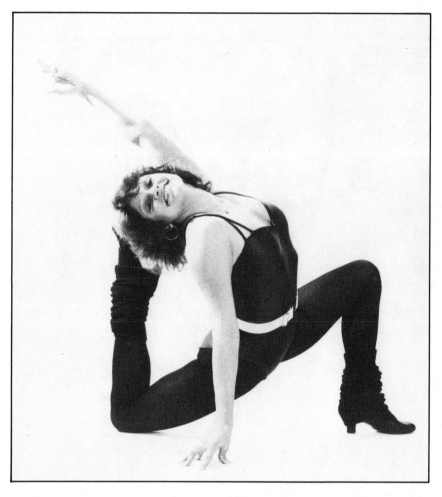

Exercise	Muscle/Area Stretched
1. Cannonball	Low Back, Neck Extensors
2. Spread Eagle	Groin
3. Figure Four	Hamstrings
4. Pretzel	Trunk Rotators, Neck Rotators
5. Altar Boy	Quadriceps, Shins
6. Pillar	Biceps, Latissimus, Wrist Flexors

TABLE 4-5. Specific stretches for dance.

FOOTBALL

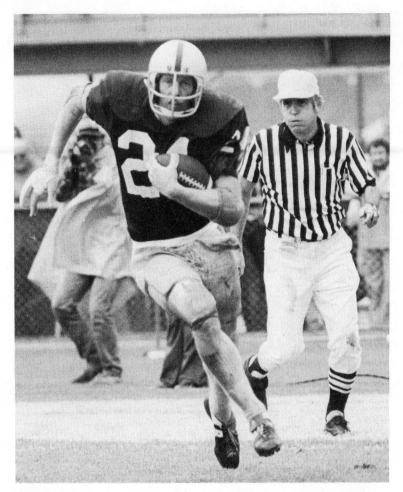

Exercises	Muscle/Area Stretched
1. Cannonball	Low Back, Neck Extensors
2. Spread Eagle	Groin
3. Figure Four	Hamstrings
4. Pretzel	Trunk Rotators, Neck Rotators
5. Fencer	Hip Flexors
6. Airplane	Chest

TABLE 4-6. Specific stretches for football.

GOLF

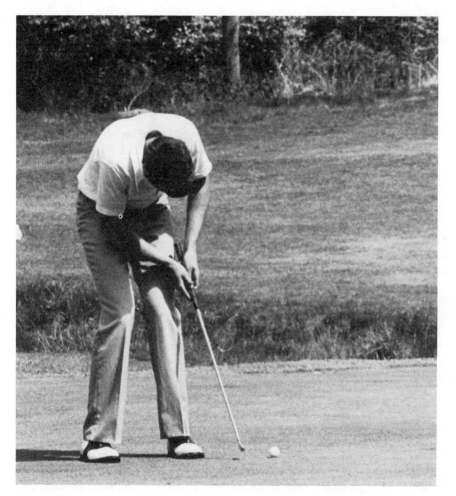

Exercises	Muscle/Area Stretched
1. Pillar	Biceps, Latissimus, Wrist Flexors
2. Teacup	Rib Cage, Neck Flexors
3. Fencer	Hip Flexors
4. Cannonball	Low Back, Neck Extensors
5. Criss Cross	Hip Rotators, Trunk Rotators
6. Pretzel	Trunk Rotators, Neck Rotators

TABLE 4-7. Specific stretches for golf.

JOGGING

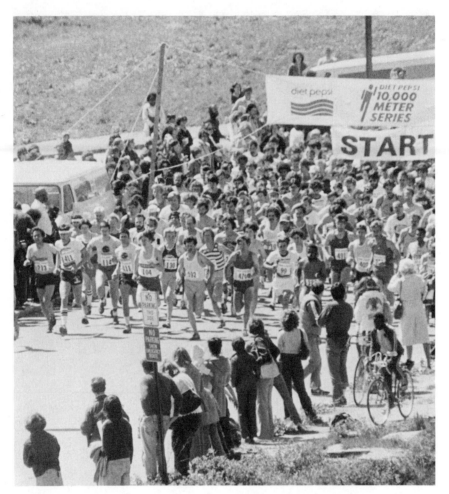

Exercises	Muscle/Area Stretched
1. Leaning Tower	Calves
2. Fencer	Hip Flexors
3. Altar Boy	Quadriceps, Shins
4. Cannonball	Low Back, Neck Extensors
5. Can Opener	Low Back, Hip Extensors
6. Figure Four	Hamstrings

TABLE 4-8. Specific stretches for jogging.

KARATE

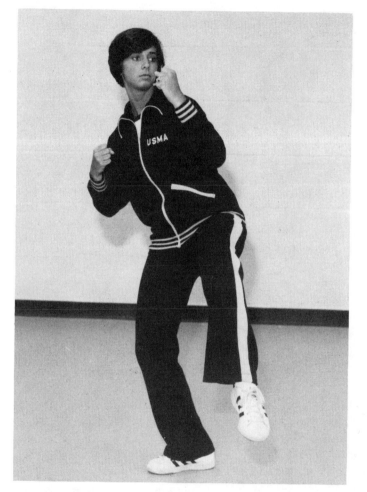

Exercises	Muscle/Area Stretched
1. Cannonball	Low Back, Neck Extensors
2. Spread Eagle	Groin
3. Figure Four	Hamstrings
4. Pretzel	Trunk Rotators, Neck Rotators
5. Altar Boy	Quadriceps, Shins
6. Fencer	Hip Flexors

TABLE 4-9. Specific stretches for karate.

RACQUETBALL/SQUASH

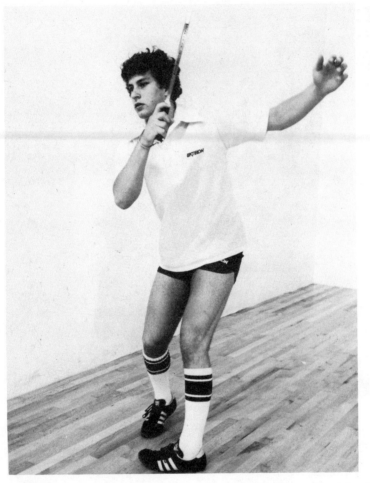

Exercises	Muscle/Area Stretched
1 Spread Eagle	Groin
2. Figure Four	Hamstrings
3. Airplane	Chest
4. Pillar	Biceps, Latissimus, Wrist Flexors
5. Chicken Wing	Triceps
6. Leaning Tower	Calves

TABLE 4-10. Specific stretches for racquetball and squash.

SKIING

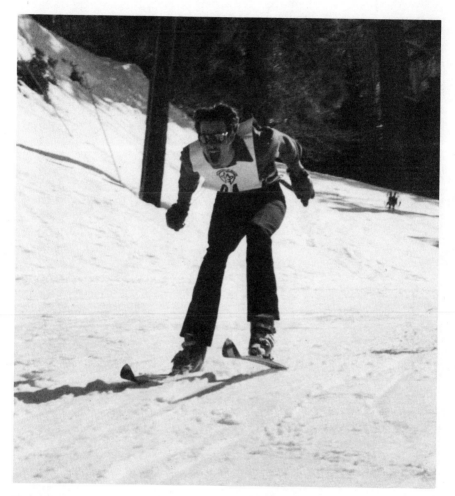

Exercises	Muscle/Area Stretched
1. Leaning Tower	Calves
2. Altar Boy	Quadriceps, Shins
3. Figure Four	Hamstrings
4. Spread Eagle	Groin
5. Pretzel	Trunk Rotators, Neck Rotators
6. Cannonball	Low Back, Neck Extensors

TABLE 4-11. Specific stretches for skiing.

SOCCER

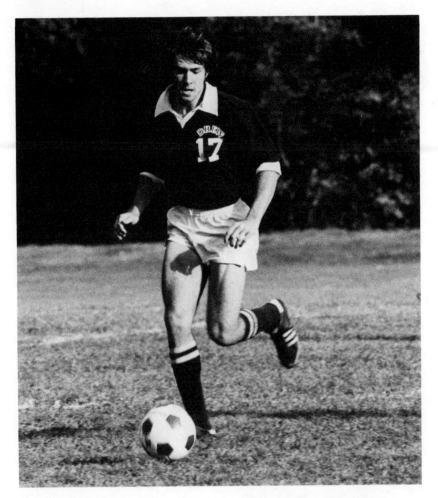

Exercises	Muscle/Area Stretched
1. Cannonball	Low Back, Neck Extensors
2. Spread Eagle	Groin
3. Figure Four	Hamstrings
4. Altar Boy	Quadriceps, Shins
5. Fencer	Hip Flexors
6. Leaning Tower	Calves

TABLE 4-12. Specific stretches for soccer.

SWIMMING/ROWING

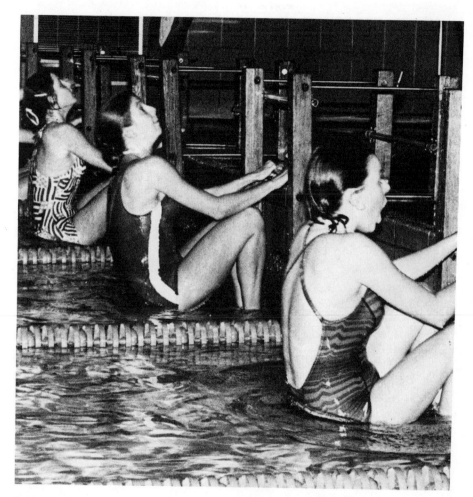

Exercises	Muscle/Area Stretched
1. Pillar	Biceps, Latissimus, Wrist Flexors
2. Chicken Wing	Triceps
3. Airplane	Chest
4. Twine	Shoulder Rotators
5. Windshield Wipers	Neck Rotators
6. Altar Boy	Quadriceps, Shins

TABLE 4-13. Specific stretches for swimming and rowing.

TENNIS

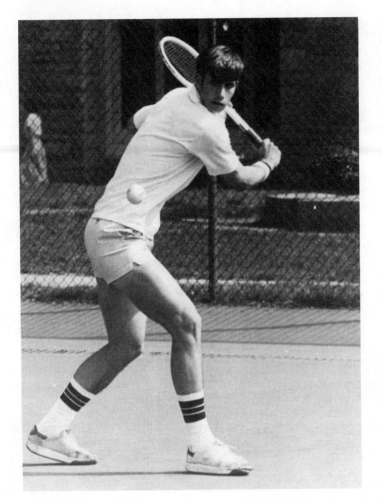

Exercises	Muscle/Area Stretched
1. Spread Eagle	Groin
2. Figure Four	Hamstrings
3. Airplane	Chest
4. Pillar	Biceps, Latissimus, Wrist Flexors
5. Chicken Wing	Triceps
6. Leaning Tower	Calves

TABLE 4-14. Specific stretches for tennis.

VOLLEYBALL

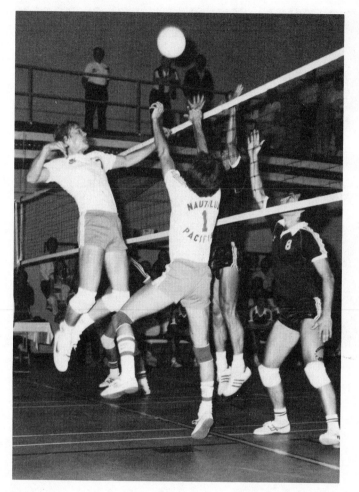

Exercises	Muscle/Area Stretched
1. Leaning Chair	Wrist Flexors
2. Figure Four	Hamstrings
3. Spread Eagle	Groin
4. Fencer	Hip Flexors
5. Pillar	Biceps, Latissimus, Wrist Flexors
6. Leaning Tower	Calves

TABLE 4-15. Specific stretches for volleyball.

WRESTLING

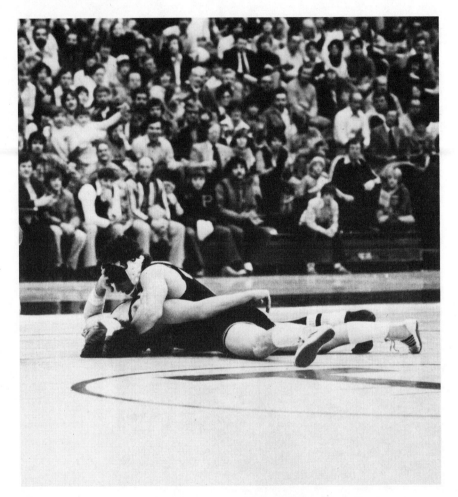

Exercises	Muscle/Area Stretched
1. Cannonball	Low Back, Neck Extensors
2. Pretzel	Trunk Rotators, Neck Rotators
3. Spread Eagle	Groin
4. Teacup	Rib Cage, Neck Flexors
5. Pillar	Biceps, Latissimus, Wrist Flexors
6. Airplane	Chest

TABLE 4-16. Specific stretches for wrestling.

SPORT STRETCHES

AIRPLANE (Chest)

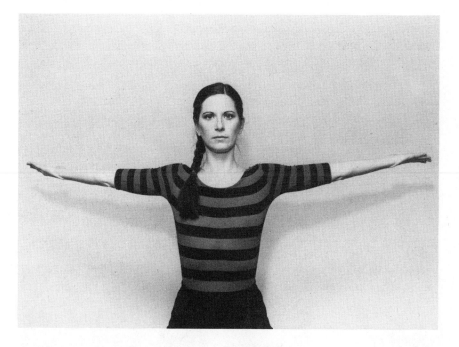

Stand with your arms straight out and at shoulder height. Turn your palms up, and slowly pull your arms back.

*This section presents in alphabetical order the sixteen recommended specific sport stretches. The eleven Fundamental Stretch exercises are included.

ALTAR BOY (Quadriceps, Shins)

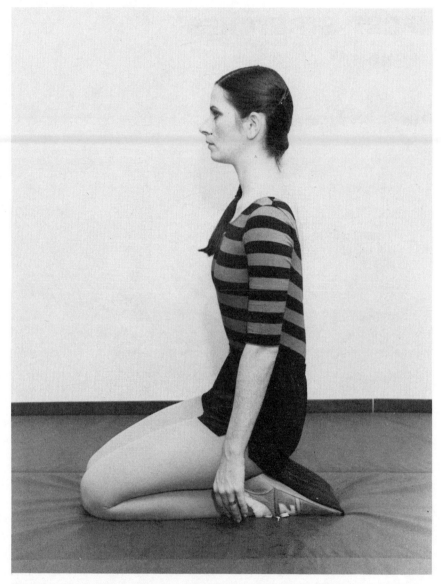

Kneel with the tops of your feet flat on the floor. Slowly sit back on
your heels.
*Note: If you have knee problems, don't bend your knees into this
position.

CANNONBALL (Low Back, Neck Extensors)

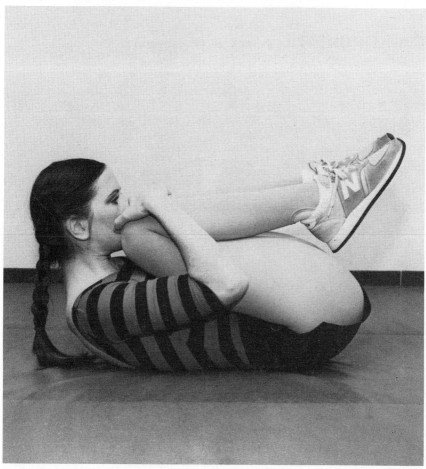

Lie flat on your back. Bend your knees, and place your feet flat on the floor. Grab your knees with your hands, and slowly pull your knees to your chest. At the same time, curl your head to your knees.

CAN OPENER (Low Back, Hip Extensors)

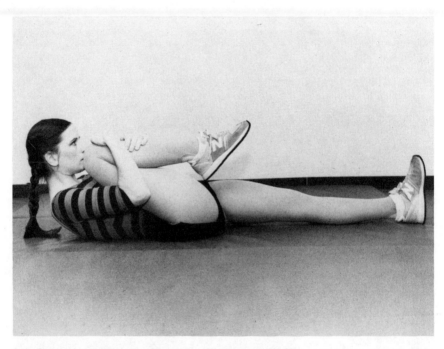

Lie flat on your back. Slowly pull your right knee to your chest with your hands. Repeat with the other leg.

CHICKEN WING (Triceps)

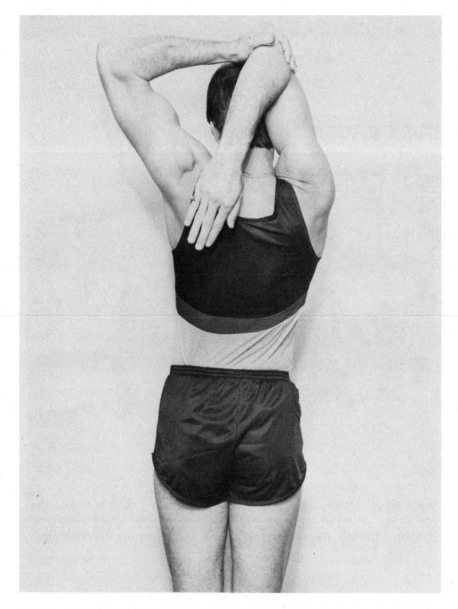

Stand with your right arm bent behind your head. Grasp your right elbow with your left hand, and slowly pull the elbow away from your head. Reverse arm positions, and stretch your other arm.

CRISS CROSS (Hip Rotators, Trunk Rotators)

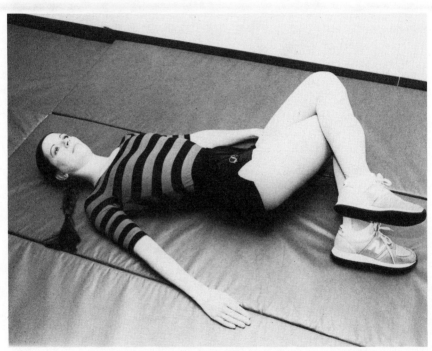

Lie flat on your back. Bend your knees, and place your feet flat on the floor. Cross your left leg over your right leg. Slowly lower both legs together to the left. Reverse leg positions, and stretch to the other side.

FENCER (Hip Flexor)

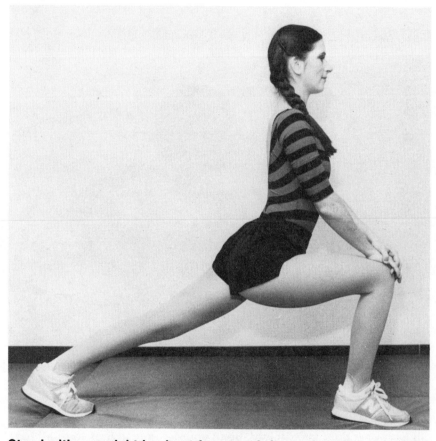

Stand with your right leg bent far enough forward so that your right knee is directly over your right ankle. Straighten your left leg, and raise it on the ball of your left foot. Slowly lower your hips, keeping your back straight. Reverse leg positions, and stretch the other leg.

FIGURE FOUR (Hamstrings)

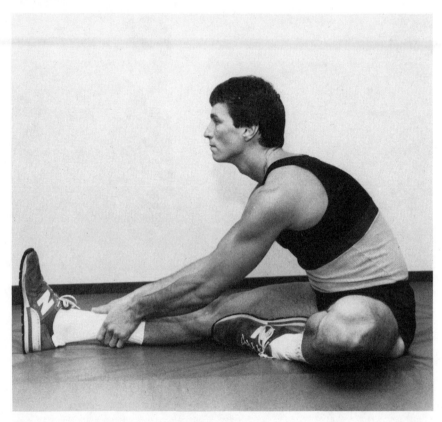

Sit with your right leg straight. Bend your left leg so that your left foot slightly touches the inside of the right thigh. Slowly bend forward at the hips, and try to touch your chin to your right foot. Then reverse leg positions, and repeat the stretch.

LEANING CHAIR (Wrist Flexors)

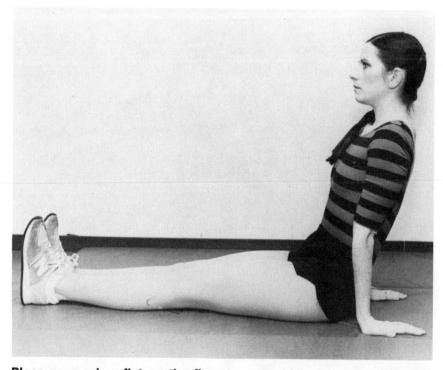

Place your palms flat on the floor to your sides. Point your thumbs outward and your fingers backward. Straighten your elbows. Then slowly lean back.

LEANING TOWER A (Calves)

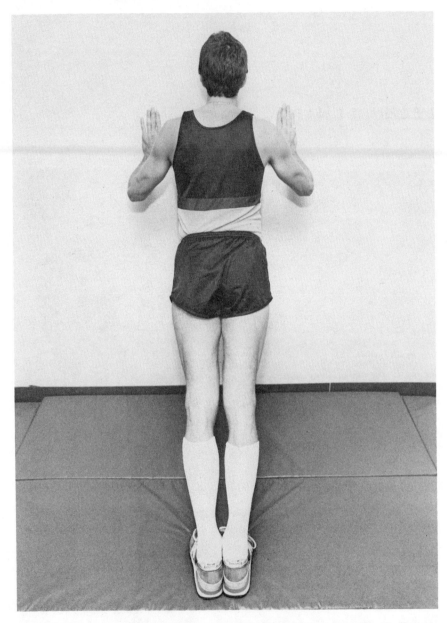

a) Stand facing a wall. Straighten your legs, and place your heels flat on the floor. Using your arms for support, slowly lean forward at the hips.

LEANING TOWER B (Calves)

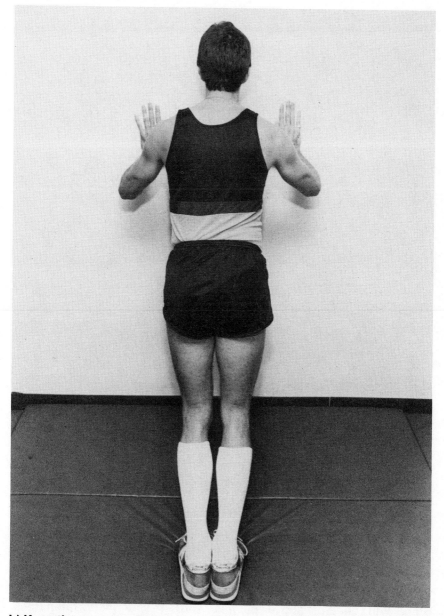

b) Keep the same position as in a. But instead of your hips, slowly bend forward at the knees. Be sure to keep your heels flat on the floor.

PILLAR (Biceps, Latissimus, Wrist Flexors)

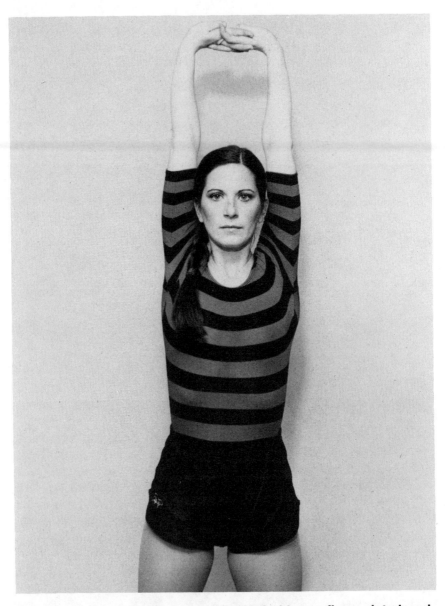

Stand with your arms above your head and with your fingers interlaced. Straighten your arms, then turn your palms forward and up. Slowly pull your arms back.

PRETZEL (Trunk Rotators, Neck Rotators)

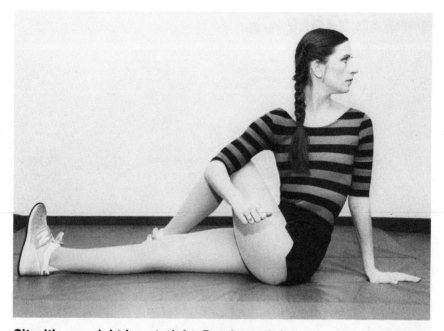

Sit with your right leg straight. Bend your left leg over your right leg, and rest your left foot flat on the floor on the outside of your right knee. Touch your right elbow to the outside of your left knee. Place your left hand on the floor behind you. Then slowly look over your left shoulder, and rotate your trunk to the left. At the same time, apply counter-pressure with your right elbow against your left knee. Reverse leg positions, and stretch to the other side.

SPREAD EAGLE (Groin)

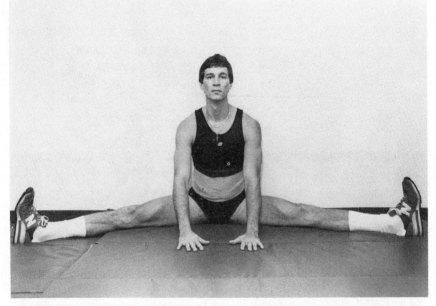

Sit with your legs spread wide. Slowly lean forward, keeping your legs straight.

TEACUP (Rib Cage, Neck Flexors)

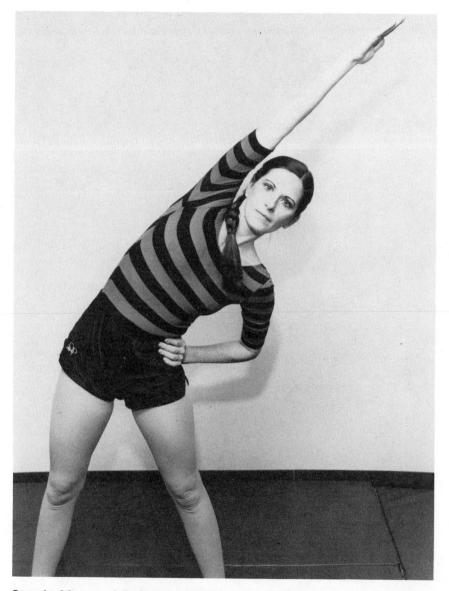

Stand with your right hand straight above your head and with your left hand resting on your left hip. Slowly bend to your left, and pull your right arm over your head. Reverse arm positions, and stretch to the other side.

TWINE (Shoulder Rotators)

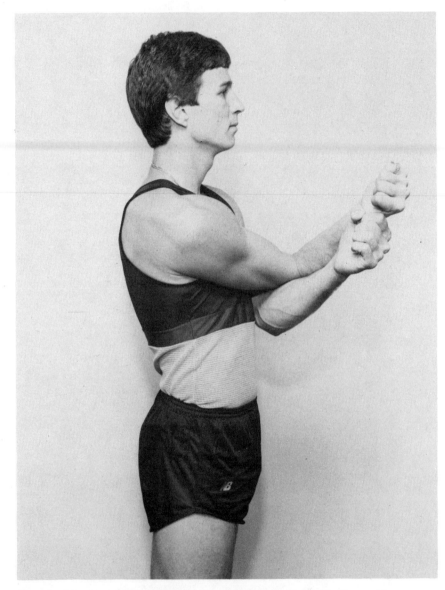

Stand with your right arm bent at a 90° angle in front of you. Turn your right palm toward your stomach. Bend your left arm underneath your right arm, and grasp your right thumb with your left hand. Slowly pull your right arm down to the floor.

WINDSHIELD WIPERS (Neck Rotators)

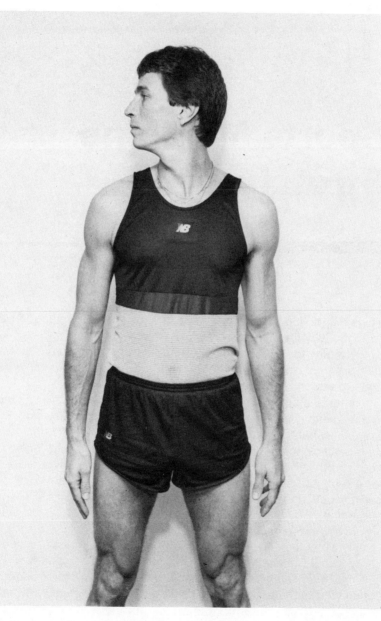

Slowly turn your head to the right, and look over your right shoulder. Repeat to the other side.

5

Sports Medicine Stretches

It wasn't too long ago that athletic injuries meant long periods of rest and inactivity for otherwise healthy athletes.

Not any more. Today's sportsmedicine experts prescribe aggressive programs of exercise to rehabilitate injured athletes, returning them to action faster and stronger than ever.

Injured athletes who refrain from activities eventually will recover. In the meantime, they lose the flexibility and conditioning they've worked so hard to develop. Once their injuries have healed, athletes then must retrain their bodies, slowly returning them to a level of competitive fitness. All too often, however, eager players ignore the need for a reconditioning period. They immediately resume their activities and expect top performances from unstretched muscles, ligaments, and tendons.

What happens? Athletes wind up reinjured.

The problem in such cases begins when the injuries first occur. No injury should prevent a player from keeping fit, for athletes should continue exercising during periods of rehabilitation. In sportsmedicine centers throughout the world, athletes are encouraged to maintain their conditioning with programs such as the Fundamental Stretch. Athletes are also given specific exercises designed to strengthen their injury sites.

During rehabilitation, players may have to refrain from participating in sports. As they heal, they still exercise. Once the athletes are ready for competition, they return in peak condition and with fewer risks of reinjury.

The sportsmedicine stretches described in this chapter are ideal for treating athletic injuries. Each injury listed includes three stretches, developed as rehabilitation for particular muscle groups. For the best results, perform the stretches five times each, holding all stretches for ten seconds. This routine should be undertaken three times daily until your injury is completely healed and pain free.

All the injuries defined are located on the right side of the body. Should you injure your left side, just reverse the positions of the stretches.

Two reminders. First, don't diagnose your own injury. If you hurt yourself, allow a qualified physician to make that diagnosis for you. Then show your physician the sportsmedicine stretches recommended in this book, and work together to develop a rehabilitation program best suited for you.

Second, and most importantly, don't neglect the rest of your body as you exercise your injury back to health. Make a daily commitment to the Fundamental Stretch, and you'll return to your sport in top form.

BICIPITAL TENDONITIS

- inflammation and pain along the biceps tendon, located in the front of the shoulder.

- caused by overuse in such activities as throwing, rowing, and swimming.

Bicipital Tendonitis Exercise No. 1

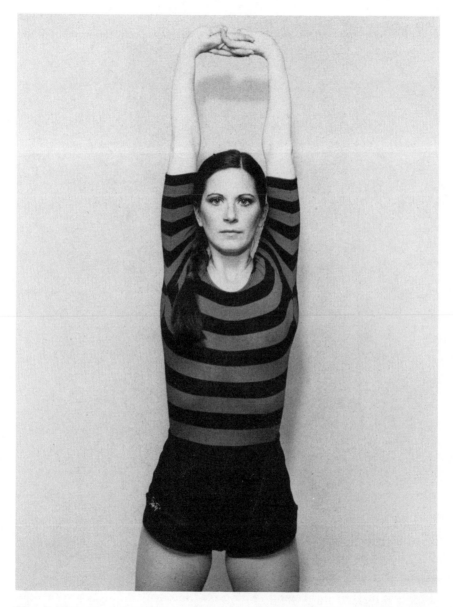

Stand with your arms above your head and with your fingers interlaced. Straighten your arms, then turn your palms forward and up. Slowly pull your arms back.

Bicipital Tendonitis Exercise No. 2

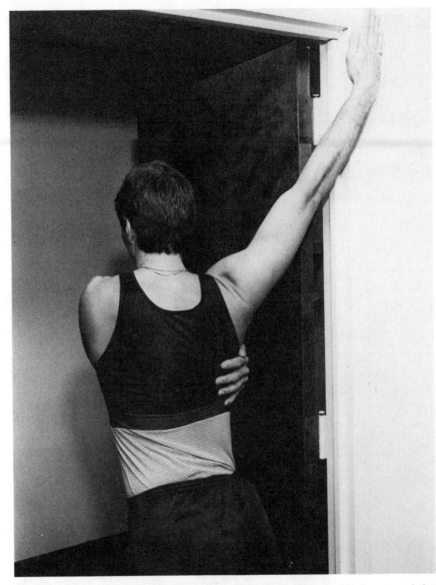

Stand with your right hand resting on the doorjamb. Keep your right arm straight. Grasp the right side of your rib cage with your left hand, and slowly lean forward through the doorway. At the same time, pull your trunk to your left.

Bicipital Tendonitis Exercise No. 3

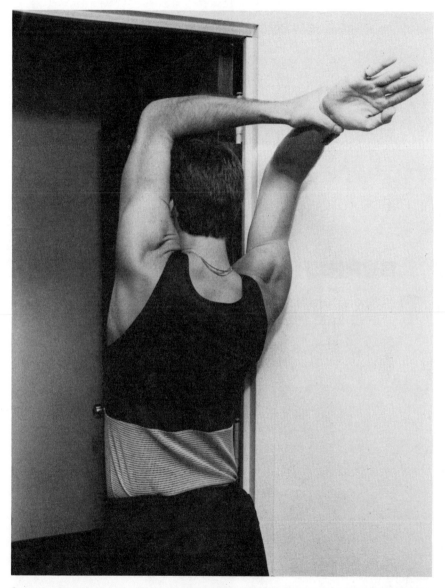

Stand with the back of your right upper arm flat against the doorjamb. Bend your left arm behind your head, and grasp your right wrist with your left hand. Slowly lean forward through the doorway. At the same time, push your right hand away from your head.

BURNER

- neck pain extending from the base of the skull into the shoulders and upper back.

- caused by a head tackle in football.

Burner Exercise No. 1

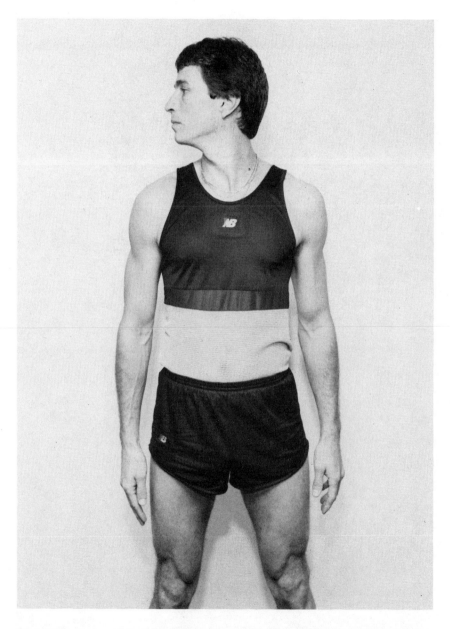

Slowly turn your head to the right, and look over your right shoulder.
Repeat to the other side.

Burner Exercise No. 2

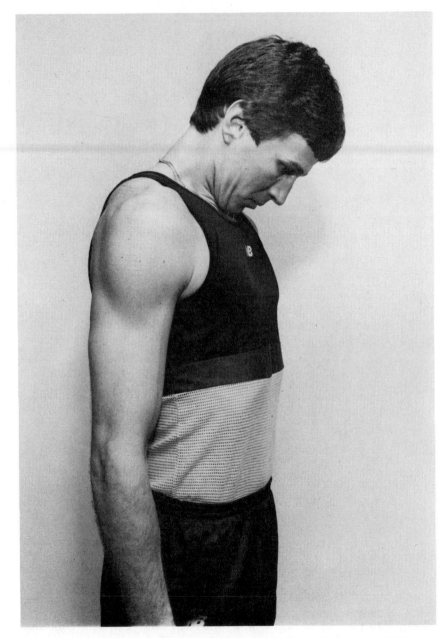

Slowly bend your head forward, and touch your chin to your chest.

Burner Exercise No. 3

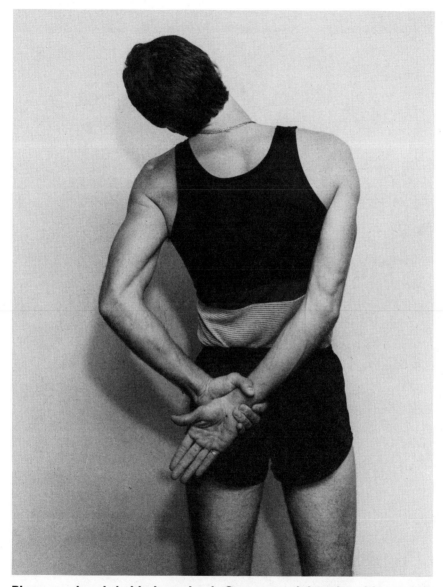

Place your hands behind your back. Grasp your right wrist with your left hand. Slowly pull your right arm to your left. At the same time, try to touch your left ear to your left shoulder. Reverse arm positions, and stretch to the other side.

CHARLEY HORSE

- pain and tightness in the quadriceps (front thigh) muscle.

- caused by a direct blow to the thigh.

Charley Horse Exercise No. 1

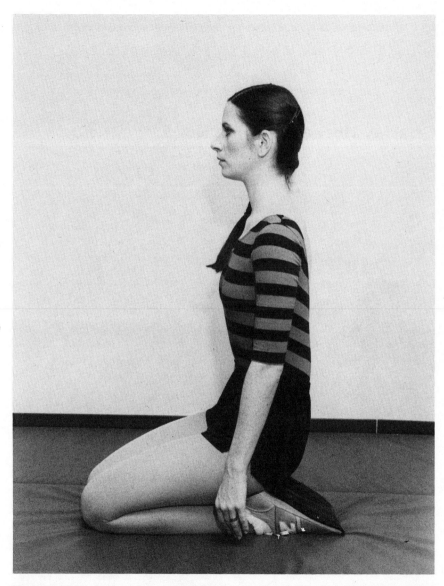

Kneel with the tops of your feet flat on the floor. Slowly sit back on your heels.

*NOTE: If you have knee problems, don't bend your knees into this position.

Charley Horse Exercise No. 2

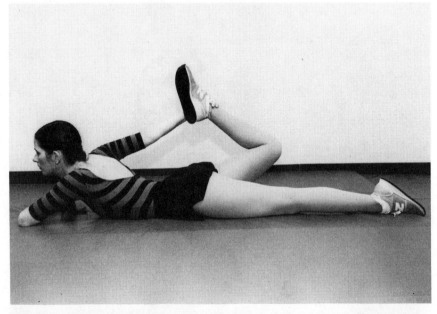

Lie on your stomach. Bend your right knee, and try to touch your right heel to your right buttock. Next, grasp your right ankle with your right hand. Slowly pull your ankle toward the back of your head. Avoid twisting your trunk.

Charley Horse Exercise No. 3

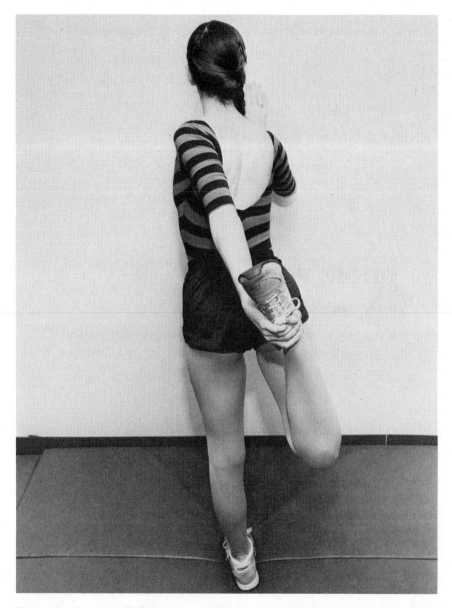

Stand facing a wall. Bend your right knee, and try to touch your right heel to your right buttock. Grasp your right ankle with your left hand. Slowly pull your ankle toward the back of your head.

GROIN PULL

- tenderness along the inner thigh.
- caused by activities which involve changing directions while running, e.g., tennis, soccer, and basketball.

Groin Pull Exercise No. 1

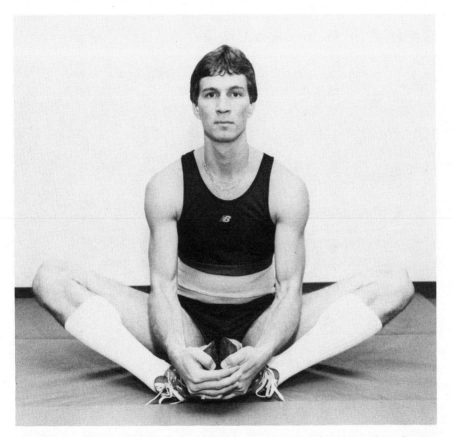

Sit with your knees bent and with the soles of your feet together. Grasp your toes with both hands. Slowly pull your heels toward your groin. Use your hip muscles to slowly push your knees to the floor.

Groin Pull Exercise No. 2

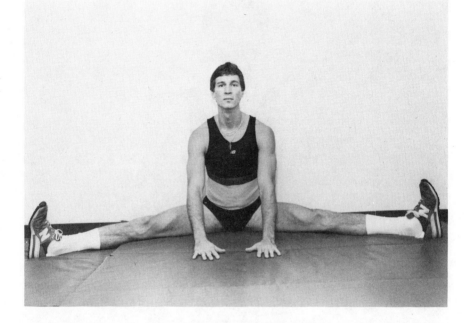

Sit with your legs spread wide. Slowly lean forward, keeping your legs straight.

Groin Pull Exercise No. 3

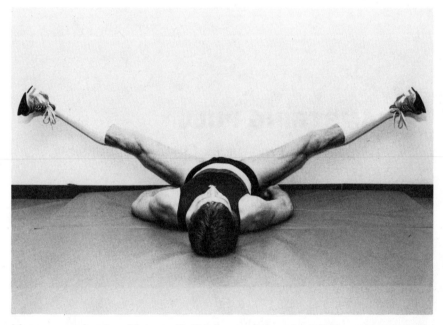

Lie on your back with your buttocks and your feet flat against a wall. Keep your legs straight and your heels on the wall. Then slowly slide your legs apart.

HAMSTRING PULL

- tenderness in the back of the thigh, possibly extending up to the buttocks.

- caused by inadequate warm-ups or by poor body mechanics in running sports.

Hamstring Pull Exercise No. 1

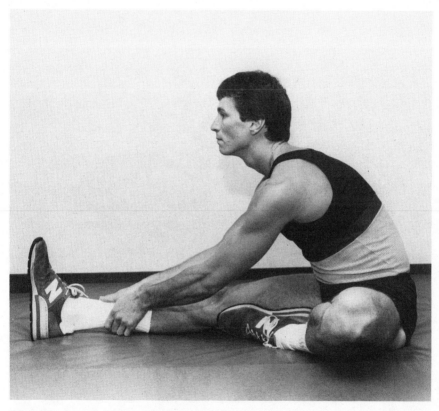

Sit with your right leg straight. Bend your left leg so that your left foot slightly touches the inside of the right thigh. Slowly bend forward at the hips, and try to touch your chin to your right foot.

Hamstring Pull Exercise No. 2

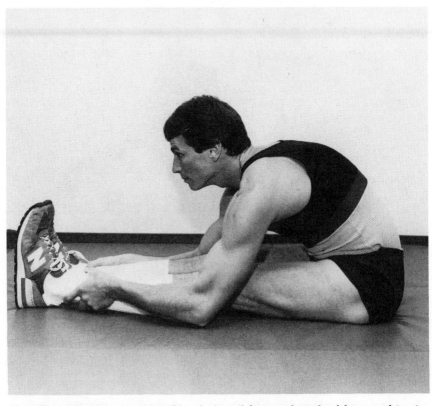

Sit with your legs straight. Slowly bend forward at the hips, and try to touch your chin to your toes.

Hamstring Pull Exercise No. 3

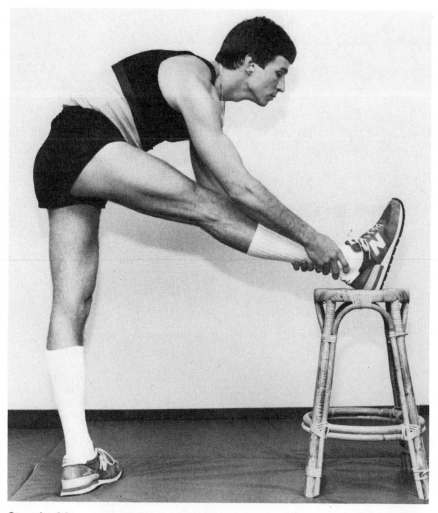

Stand with your right heel resting on a table, stool, or chair (comfortable height). Straighten your right leg. Slowly bend forward at the hips, and try to touch your chin to your toes.

HIP POINTER

- pain and tenderness along the iliac crest (hip bone).

- caused by a direct blow to the hip, as in contact sports.

Hip Pointer Exercise No. 1

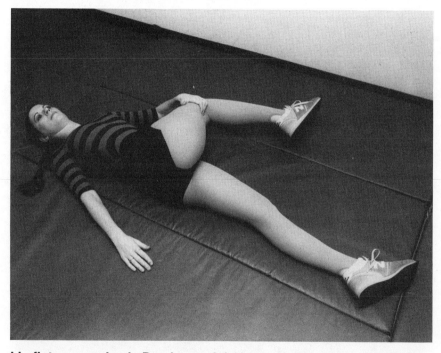

Lie flat on your back. Bend your right knee to your chest, then slowly move it to the left side of your body. Grasp just above the right knee with your left hand. Keep your shoulders flat on the floor, and slowly push your right knee to the floor.

Hip Pointer Exercise No. 2

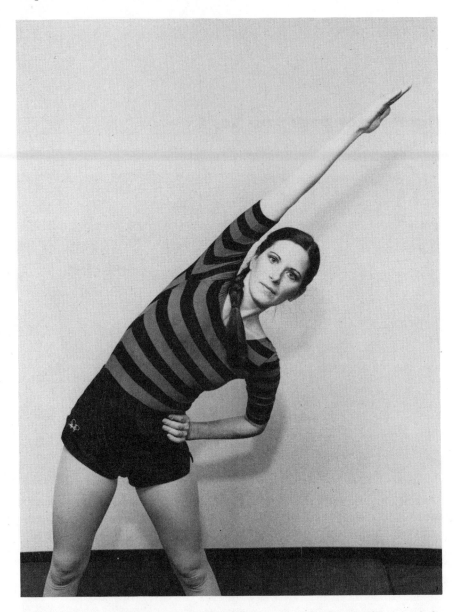

Stand with your right hand straight above your head and with your left hand resting on your left hip. Slowly bend to your left, and pull your right arm over your head.

Hip Pointer Exercise No. 3

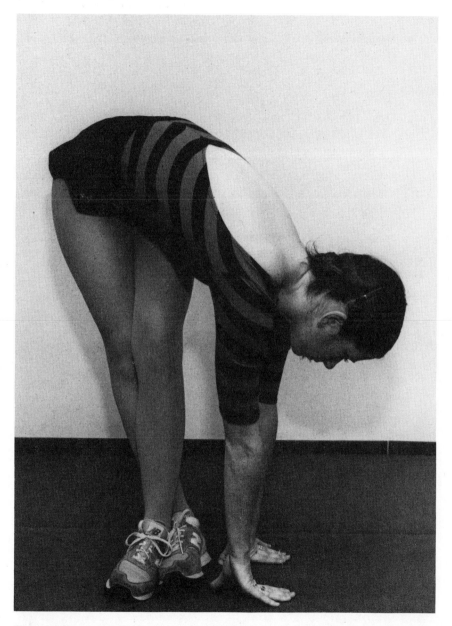

Stand with your right leg crossed behind your left leg. Rotate your trunk
to the left. Then slowly bend over, and reach for the floor.

LOW BACK STRAIN

- tenderness and lack of motion in the low back region.

- caused by improper body mechanics, by inadequate warm-ups, or by overuse of the erector spinae (low back) muscles.

Low Back Strain Exercise No. 1

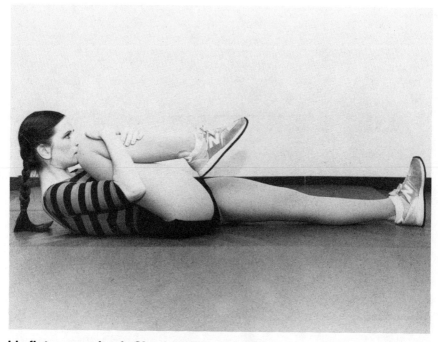

Lie flat on your back. Slowly pull your right knee to your chest with your hands. Repeat with the other leg.

Low Back Strain Exercise No. 2

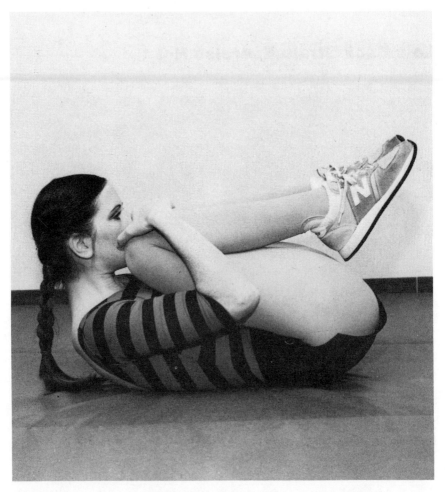

Lie flat on your back. Bend your knees, and place your feet flat on the floor. Grab your knees with your hands, and slowly pull your knees to your chest. At the same time, curl your head to your knees.

Low Back Strain Exercise No. 3

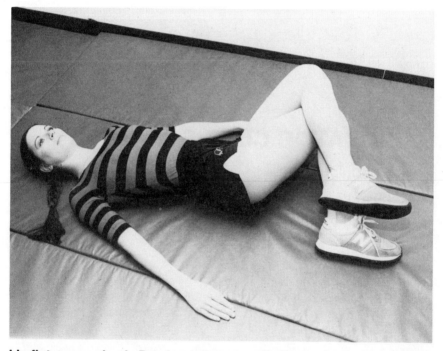

Lie flat on your back. Bend your knees, and place your feet flat on the floor. Cross your left leg over your right leg. Slowly lower both legs together to the left. Reverse leg positions, and stretch to the other side.

ROTATOR CUFF STRAIN

- shoulder pain.

- caused by a fall onto an outstretched arm or by improper throwing techniques.

Rotator Cuff Strain Exercise No. 1

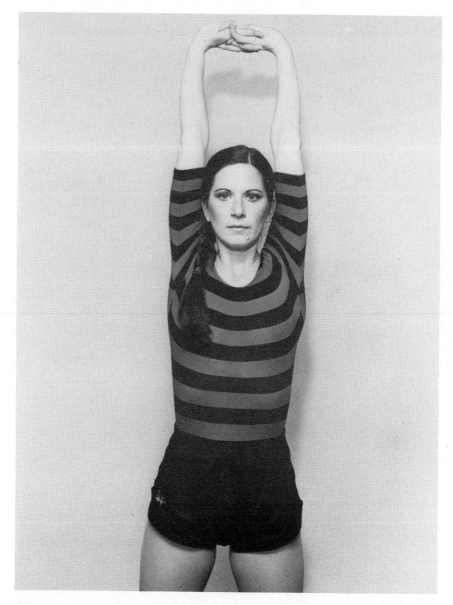

Stand with your arms above your head and with your fingers interlaced. Straighten your arms, then turn your palms forward and up. Slowly pull your arms back.

Rotator Cuff Strain Exercise No. 2

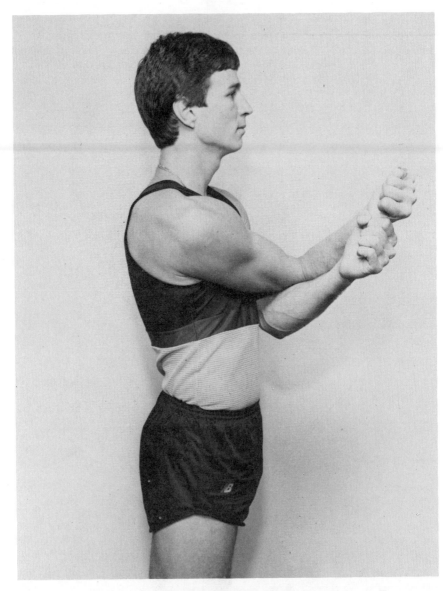

Stand with your right arm bent at a 90° angle in front of you. Turn your right palm toward your stomach. Bend your left arm underneath your right arm, and grasp your right thumb with your left hand. Slowly pull your right arm down to the floor.

Rotator Cuff Strain Exercise No. 3

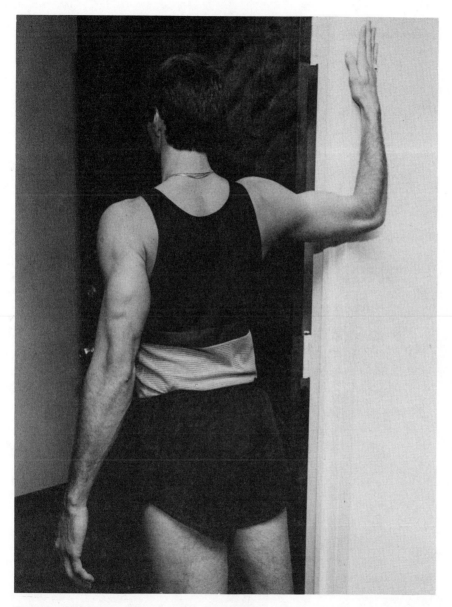

Stand with the inside of your right upper arm against the doorjamb. Your elbow should be at shoulder level and bent at a right angle. Slowly lean forward through the doorway.

SHIN SPLINTS

- tenderness along the tibia (shin).

- caused by wearing improper footwear, by running activities, or by inadequate warm-ups.

Shin Splints Exercise No. 1

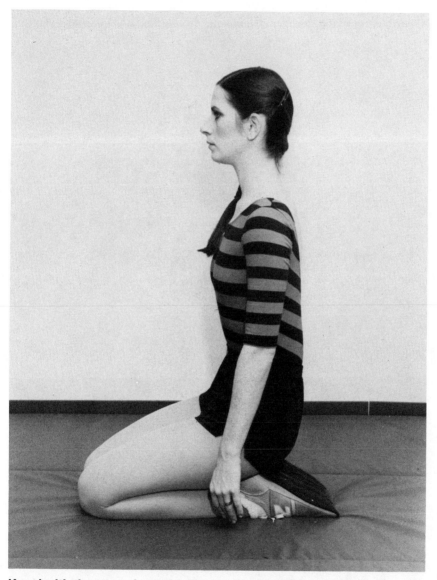

Kneel with the tops of your feet flat on the floor. Slowly sit back on your heels.

*NOTE: If you have knee problems, don't bend your knees into this position.

Shin Splints Exercise No. 2

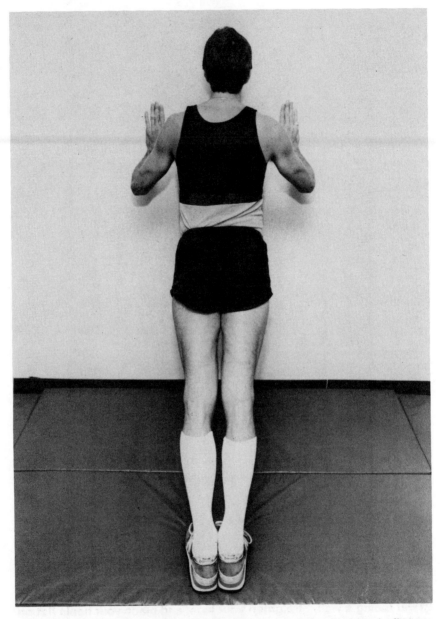

Stand facing a wall. Straighten your legs, and place your heels flat on the floor. Using your arms for support, slowly lean forward at the hips.

Shin Splints Exercise No. 3

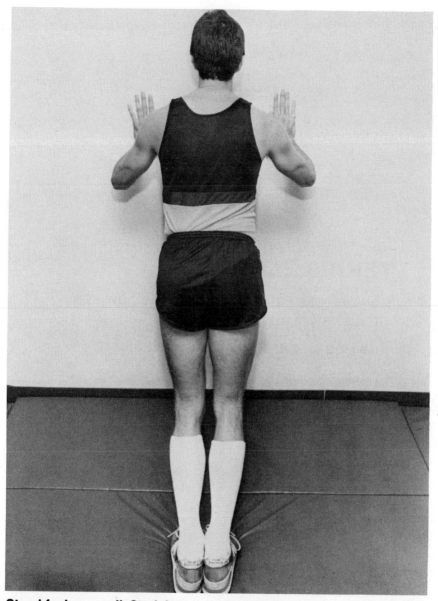

Stand facing a wall. Straighten your legs, and place your heels flat on the floor. Using your arms for support, slowly bend forward at the knees.

TENNIS ELBOW

- tenderness extending from the elbow into the forearm and wrist.

- caused by the stroke in racquet sports.

Tennis Elbow Exercise No. 1

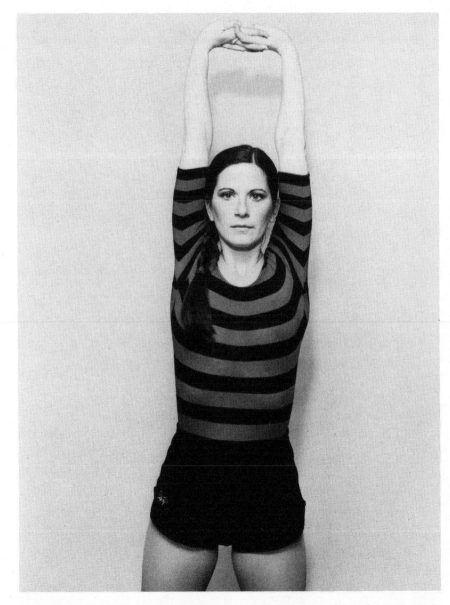

Stand with your arms above your head and with your fingers interlaced. Straighten your arms, then turn your palms forward and up. Slowly pull your arms back.

Tennis Elbow Exercise No. 2

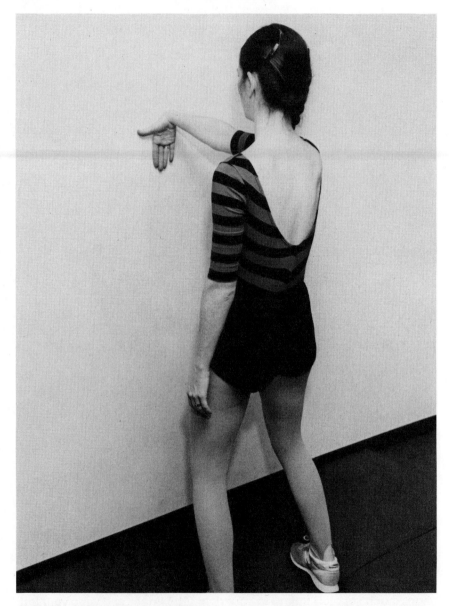

Stand facing a wall. Place the back of your right hand flat against the wall. Point your thumb to the left and your other fingers downward. Straighten your right elbow. Slowly lean down.

Tennis Elbow Exercise No. 3

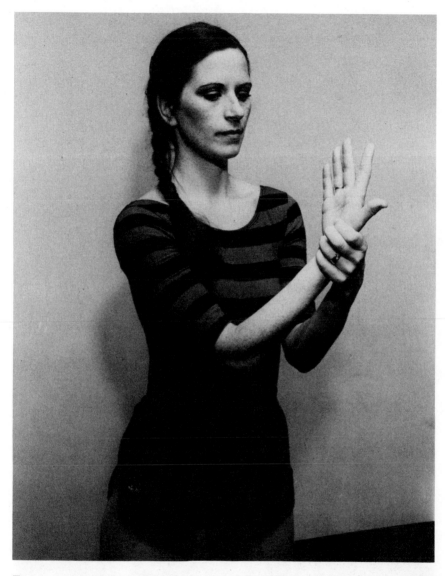

Turn up your right palm. Place your left hand underneath your right hand. Touch your left thumb to your right little finger, and wrap your left fingers around the base of your right thumb. Slowly rotate your right hand outward by pushing with your left thumb and pulling with your left fingers.

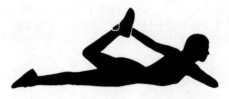

Spontaneous Stretches

Stretching can be done anytime or anywhere. It takes so little effort to gain so many benefits. Whether you're sitting, walking, supine or standing, there's always room for a good, productive stretch.

Each of the exercises you see in this chapter works a specific muscle group. Although all the exercises can be performed spontaneously, don't rush them. Follow the stretching strategy, and hold every stretch for ten seconds.

If you prefer to work muscles that aren't included in one of the spontaneous stretches, find an exercise elsewhere in this book that satisfies your muscle stretch needs. Then modify the exercise so that it can be used as a spontaneous stretch.

LOW BACK

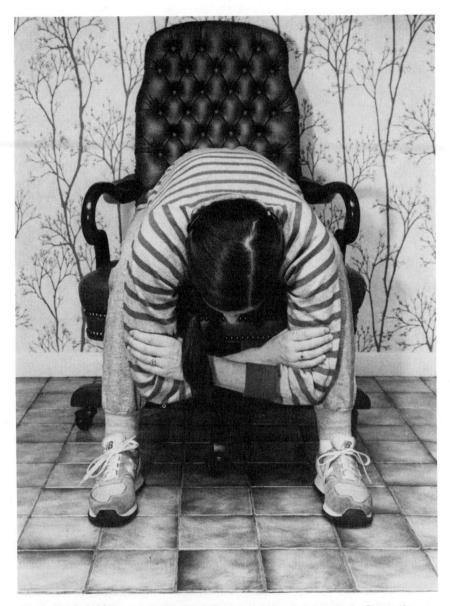

You can stretch your low back whenever you sit in a chair. Spread your feet apart, and grab your elbows with the opposite hands. Slowly bend forward between your legs, and try to touch your elbows to the floor.

GROIN

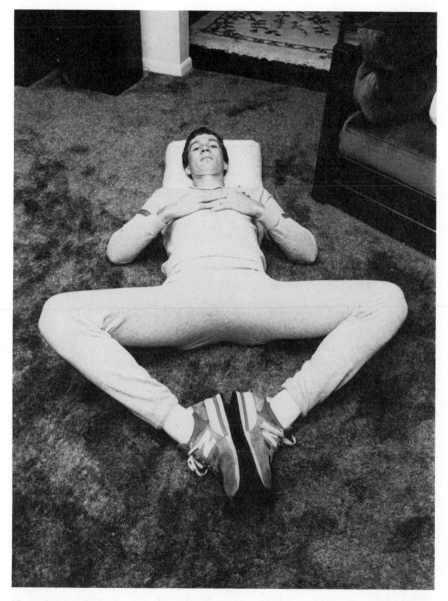

If you're lying down, you can stretch your groin muscles by rolling over on your back and placing the soles of your feet together. Use your hip muscles to slowly push your knees to the floor.

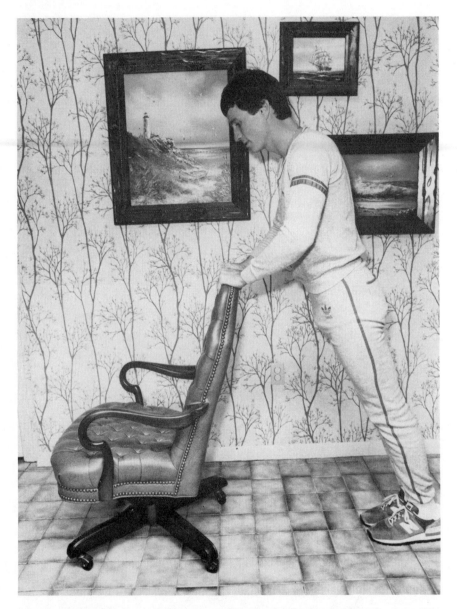

Near a curb? Then stretch your calves by leaning your heels over the curb's edge. You also can do this spontaneous stretch on a stair. For better balance, hold onto a sturdy object as you perform the stretch.

ARMS AND SHOULDERS

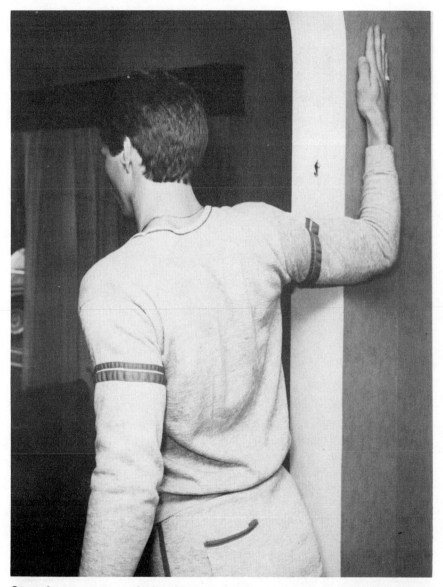

Stretch your arm and shoulder muscles as you walk through a door. Place the inside of your right upper arm against the doorjamb. Your elbow should be at shoulder level and bent at a right angle. Slowly lean forward through the doorway.

TRUNK ROTATORS

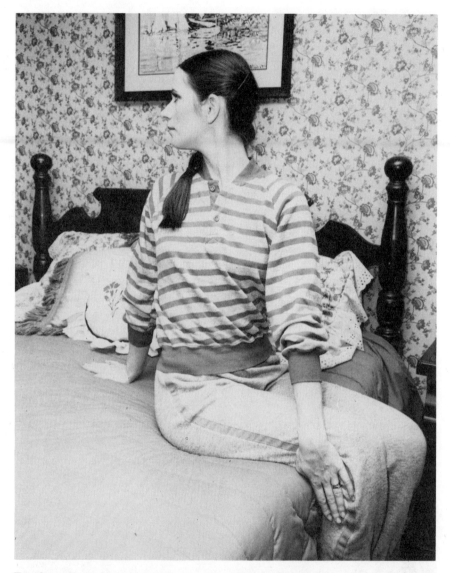

Trunk rotators love a good morning stretch. Sit on the side of the bed, and place your feet flat on the floor. Keep your legs together. Put your left hand on your right knee and your right hand behind you on the bed. Slowly look over your right shoulder, and twist your trunk to the right as far as you can. Then reverse hand positions, and twist to the left.

CHEST

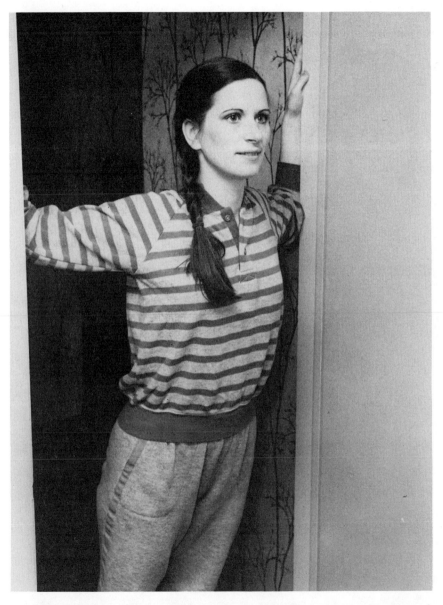

Another good doorway stretch involves spreading your arms outward at shoulder height. Place your arms against the walls on either side of the door. Then slowly lean through the doorway.

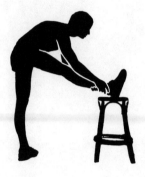

7

Muscle Charts

Understanding how your muscles work is a lot like driving a car. You can drive without knowing how the car engine operates, but that knowledge comes in handy when the car breaks down or if you're interested in keeping your auto in top condition.

Likewise, you can be very athletic and have no knowledge of body musculature. But for the sake of injury prevention and rehabilitation, it helps to understand what muscles you're working, where they're located, and how they connect to the rest of your body.

You don't have to become a physician or a physical therapist to acquire that knowledge. Instead, you can obtain a basic familiarity with muscles by studying the following charts. All the exercises in this book are identified according to the muscles they stretch. When you first perform an exercise, take the time to locate the muscles you're working in the charts. As you become more familiar with those muscles, you'll begin to appreciate their value to you as an athlete and in everyday living.

What you value, you take care of. And muscles cared for are less likely to be injured.

MUSCLE CHART I:
TRUNK IDENTIFICATION

BODY PART	SPECIFIC MUSCLES	ACTION
Side of Neck	Sternocleidomastoid	Neck Rotator
Back of Neck	Splenius Capitis Splenius Cervicis	Neck Extensor
Low Back	Spinalis *Longissimus } Erector Iliocostalis } Spinae	Trunk Extensor
Stomach	Rectus Abdominus	Trunk Flexor
Side of Trunk	External Obliques } Obliques Internal Obliques } Latissimus Dorsi	Trunk Rotator Shoulder Extensor
Rib Cage	Serratus Anterior	Shoulder Protractor

(* not pictured)

MUSCLE CHART II:
LOWER EXTREMITY IDENTIFICATION

BODY PART	SPECIFIC MUSCLES	ACTION
Inside of Hip	Adductor Magnus Adductor Longus } Adductors *Adductor Brevis Gracilis	Hip Adductor
Front of Hip	Iliopsoas	Hip Flexor
Back of Hip	Gluteus Maximus	Hip Extensor
Outside of Hip	Gluteus Medius	Hip Abductor
Front of Thigh	Rectus Femoris Vastus Medialis } Quadriceps Vastus Lateralis *Vastus Intermedius	Knee Extensor
Back of Thigh	Biceps Femoris Semitendinosus } Hamstrings Semimembranosus	Knee Flexor
Calf	Gastrocnemius Soleus	Ankle Extensor
Shin	Anterior Tibial Extensor Digitorum Longus Extensor Hallicis Longus	Ankle Flexor

(* not pictured)

MUSCLE CHART III:
UPPER EXTREMITY IDENTIFICATION

BODY PART	SPECIFIC MUSCLES	ACTION
Chest	Pectoralis Major Pectoralis Minor	Shoulder Adductor
Top of Shoulder	Trapezius	Shoulder Elevator
Outside of Shoulder	Deltoids *Rotator Cuff	Shoulder Abductor
Front of Arm	Biceps Brachialis	Elbow Flexor
Back of Arm	Triceps	Elbow Extensor
Front of Forearm	Flexor Carpi Radialis Flexor Carpi Ulnaris	Wrist Flexor
Back of Forearm	Extensor Carpi Radialis Longus Extensor Carpi Radialis Brevis Extensor Carpi Ulnaris	Wrist Extensor

(* not pictured)

MUSCLE CHART IV:
TRUNK — POSTERIOR VIEW

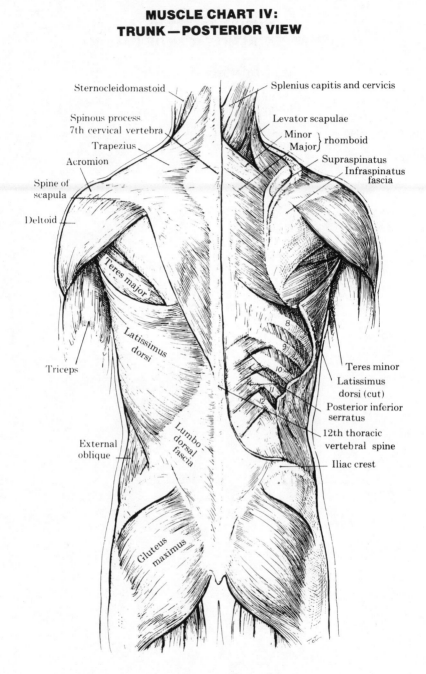

Sternocleidomastoid

Spinous process
7th cervical vertebra

Trapezius

Acromion

Spine of
scapula

Deltoid

Teres major

Latissimus
dorsi

Triceps

External
oblique

Lumbo
dorsal
fascia

Gluteus
maximus

Splenius capitis and cervicis

Levator scapulae

Minor
Major } rhomboid

Supraspinatus
Infraspinatus
fascia

8

9

10

11

12

Teres minor

Latissimus
dorsi (cut)

Posterior inferior
serratus

12th thoracic
vertebral spine

Iliac crest

(Jones and Shepard)

MUSCLE CHART V:
TRUNK — ANTERIOR VIEW

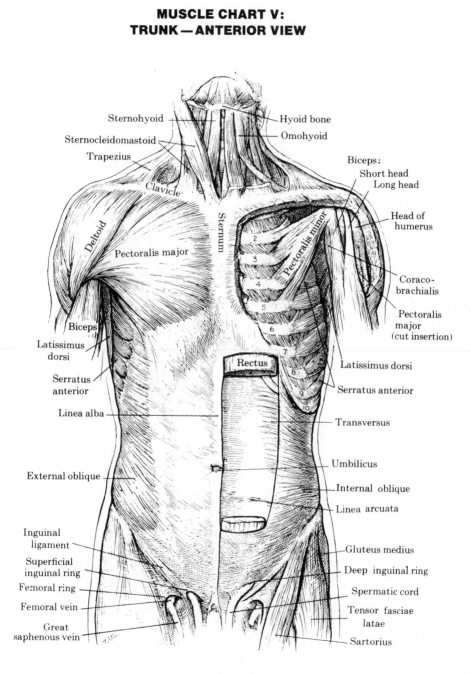

Sternohyoid

Sternocleidomastoid

Trapezius

Clavicle

Deltoid

Sternum

Pectoralis major

Biceps

Latissimus dorsi

Serratus anterior

Linea alba

External oblique

Inguinal ligament

Superficial inguinal ring

Femoral ring

Femoral vein

Great saphenous vein

Hyoid bone

Omohyoid

Biceps:
Short head
Long head

Head of humerus

Pectoralis minor

Coraco-brachialis

Pectoralis major (cut insertion)

Latissimus dorsi

Serratus anterior

Rectus

Transversus

Umbilicus

Internal oblique

Linea arcuata

Gluteus medius

Deep inguinal ring

Spermatic cord

Tensor fasciae latae

Sartorius

(Jones and Shepard)

MUSCLE CHART VI:
RIGHT LOWER EXTREMITY

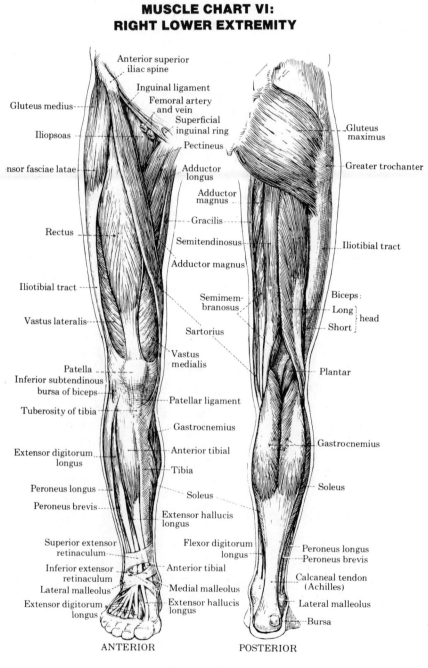

Anterior superior iliac spine

Inguinal ligament

Gluteus medius

Femoral artery and vein

Superficial inguinal ring

Iliopsoas

Pectineus

nsor fasciae latae

Adductor longus

Adductor magnus

Gracilis

Rectus

Semitendinosus

Adductor magnus

Iliotibial tract

Semimem-branosus

Vastus lateralis

Sartorius

Vastus medialis

Patella

Inferior subtendinous bursa of biceps

Tuberosity of tibia

Patellar ligament

Gastrocnemius

Extensor digitorum longus

Anterior tibial

Tibia

Peroneus longus

Soleus

Peroneus brevis

Extensor hallucis longus

Superior extensor retinaculum

Flexor digitorum longus

Inferior extensor retinaculum

Anterior tibial

Lateral malleolus

Medial malleolus

Extensor digitorum longus

Extensor hallucis longus

Gluteus maximus

Greater trochanter

Iliotibial tract

Biceps:

Long } head

Short }

Plantar

Gastrocnemius

Soleus

Peroneus longus

Peroneus brevis

Calcaneal tendon (Achilles)

Lateral malleolus

Bursa

ANTERIOR

POSTERIOR

(Jones and Shepard)

MUSCLE CHART VII:
RIGHT UPPER EXTREMITY

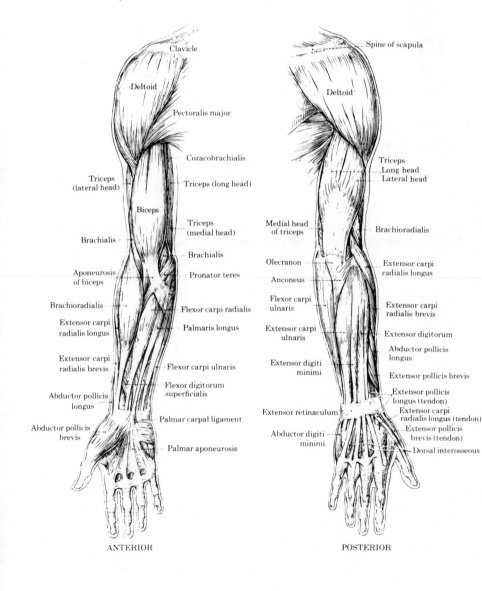

(Jones and Shepard)

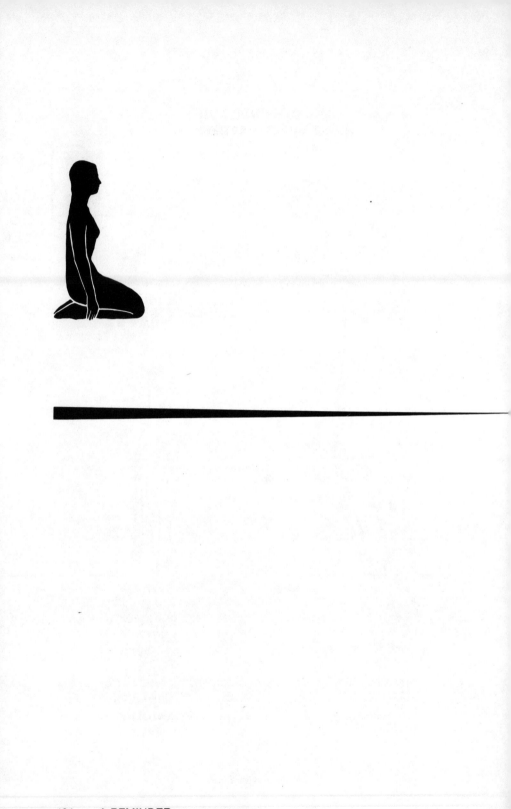

8

A Reminder

As you become accustomed to your newly acquired flexibility, don't fool yourself into thinking that you can skip your stretching exercises occasionally and still stay in shape.

Skipping a day results in lost flexibility. And a day lost cannot be regained by stretching harder another time. Once you've committed to a flexibility routine, stick with it forever if you wish to remain in top condition. Even if you give up athletics, don't give up stretching. Your muscles work for you round-the-clock. But without stretching, they don't work as well.

The following pages contain a brief reminder of the Fundamental Stretch you learned in Chapter 3. Once you're familiar with the Fundamental Stretch, use pages 126-127 as a quick overview of the exercises involved. Then perform the Fundamental Stretch everyday — wherever you are, no matter how busy you are.

Just ten minutes devoted to flexibility results in 24 hours of great muscle health.

CANNONBALL
(low back, neck extensions)

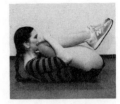

SPREAD EAGLE
(groin)

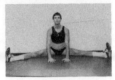

FIGURE FOUR
(hamstrings)

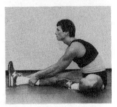

PRETZEL
(trunk rotators, neck rotators)

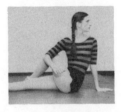

ALTAR BOY
(quadriceps, shins)

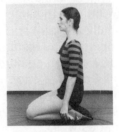

FENCER
(hip flexors)

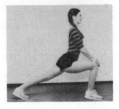

LEANING TOWER A
(calves)

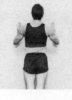

LEANING TOWER B
(calves)

AIRPLANE
(chest)

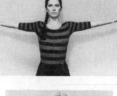

PILLAR
(biceps, latissimus, wrist flexors)

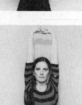

CHICKEN WING
(triceps)

TEACUP
(rib cage, neck flexors)

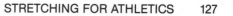

About the Author

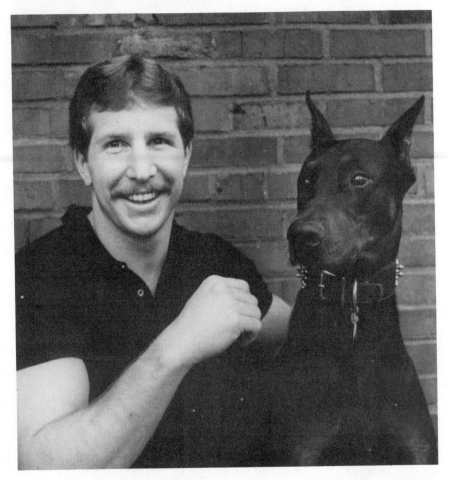

Pat Croce

presently serves as the Physical Conditioning Coach of the Philadelphia Flyers Hockey Club, Administrative Director of the Sports Medicine Clinic at Haverford Community Hospital, and President of Orthopedic and Athletic Rehabilitation.

A native of Philadelphia, Pat Croce is a cum laude graduate of the University of Pittsburgh (B.S., 1977). A Licensed Physical Therapist (LPT) and Certified Athletic Trainer (ATC), he is also an elected member of both the American College of Sports Medicine and the National Strength and Conditioning Association. As an active competitive athlete he was two-time United States National Lightweight Karate Champion.

In addition to his many appearances across the country, Pat Croce has appeared on all three major television networks and has consulted with some of the nation's finest. His previous publications in the fields of fitness and sportsmedicine are entitled *Stretch Your Life* and *Conditioning for Ice Hockey: Year Round*.